Suture like a Plastic Surgeon

Learn suturing techniques, tips & tricks from a Plastic surgeon to get the best results in surgery, emergency medicine or general practice

Hamid Tehrani

MBBS, MD, FRCS (Plast)

ISBN: 978-1-7385130-0-0

Disclaimer

The information contained within this book is for general educational purposes only. Every attempt has been made to ensure the accuracy of the contents of this book but no assurances or guarantees are given that the contents are relevant, up to date or accurate. Readers should not use any techniques or knowledge contained in this book without the prior confirmation and oversight of a trained professional.
By reading this book, the reader agrees that under no circumstances are the author, publisher or copyright holder responsible for any losses, direct or indirect, which incur as a result of the information contained within this document, including but not limited to errors, omissions or inaccuracies.

ABOUT THE AUTHOR

Mr Tehrani is the lead trainer on the Surgeryskills.com courses, responsible for training thousands of surgeons across the world. He is a Consultant Plastic, Reconstructive and Mohs Surgeon in the UK, and has a number of past and present roles including:

- UK Plastic surgery lead for the Mohs surgery specialist interest group
- UK Chair of the Skin cancer & Mohs Surgery training fellowship for Health Education England
- Lead & Chair for the National Mohs surgery MDT network
- UK lead for the surgical guidelines on Mohs surgery service standards
- Member of the Royal College of Surgeons of Edinburgh Faculty of Surgical Trainers

His research on imaging and diagnosis of Basal Cell Carcinoma led to the award of an MD degree, and he has over 50 publications in peer-reviewed journals.

In 2021 Mr Tehrani's work was recognised nationally through a Department of Health National Award for excellence in clinical practice.

He is passionate about optimising patient care and passing on his knowledge and experience through teaching and training.

CONTENTS

1 - INTRODUCTION

Suturing is a skill like so many other skills; when you see someone performing it well, it will seem effortless and easy with just a few simple steps to learn. When you actually try to suture for the first time though, it will quickly become apparent that there is more to it than meets the eye! Fortunately, as with many skills, suturing is something that can be learnt and developed with practice.

As a surgeon, our results are often judged by the scars we leave and our training is focused on constantly striving to improve and perfect our techniques. Building the correct foundations and techniques from the start are crucial to allow you to develop your skills, and this book aims to take you from the very basics through to more advanced skills, sharing tips and tricks from the field of Plastic surgery to achieve the best results you can when suturing skin.

This book assumes no knowledge of suturing whatsoever, so we will start with the very basics including the instruments used, how to handle them, and how to tie knots. We will then go on to simple suturing techniques, building up to more complex suturing as your skills improve.

All the techniques shown in this book can be performed and practiced at home, with the suture kit and materials being easily available on the internet at reasonable prices.

If you would like to develop your suturing further and see it performed in practice, you can join us on our virtual courses through our website 'Surgeryskills.com'. The courses are all pre-filmed, allowing you to take them in the comfort of your own home and at your own pace. At the end of the course, you send in a picture of some of the work you have done and you will receive personalized feedback with a certificate to confirm you have successfully completed it. The suturing course is badged by the Royal College of Surgeons of Edinburgh and BAPRAS (British Association of Plastic, Reconstructive and Aesthetic Surgeons), so it makes a very useful addition to your CV/portfolio!

Just head over to **Surgeryskills.com** to learn more.

Surgery Skills

Learn Develop Excel

2 GETTING READY TO SUTURE

While you can learn to suture by just reading this book, nothing will replace actually practicing the skills in order to improve your technique. The materials we use in this book are readily available on the internet (for example at Amazon or ebay) and are pretty reasonably priced these days. You can substitute some of the materials with household items (eg replacing a suture pad with a dish sponge, chicken thigh, etc), but as a guide your shopping list could include:

- Suture pad with pre-made 'wounds'
- Suture instrument kit, to include needle holders, toothed forceps and scissors (these kits sometimes come with a practice pad too)
- Sutures (we would suggest starting with a 3/0 silk suture on a needle that is 3/8 curved and approx. 26mm length; more on suture sizes later in the book!). Don't buy sterile sutures, just get practice ones as they are much cheaper!

It should be noted here that the term 'suture' can mean more than one thing; it is the term given to the needle and thread, the thread that has been placed to close the wound, or the process of closing the wound. The latter is also often referred to as 'stitching a wound', but it means exactly the same as 'suturing a wound'.

Suture needles come in all different shapes and sizes, many of which are used for very specific purposes, such as bowel or vascular surgery. We're going to have a look at some different types of needles and their use in skin surgery, but first let's go through the anatomy of a needle.

The needle has 3 main aspects to it, the swage, body and point (see picture). The swage is the part of the needle that attaches to the thread, the point is the tip of the needle, and the body is everything in between. The length of the needle refers to the entire length from the start of the swage to the very end of the point.

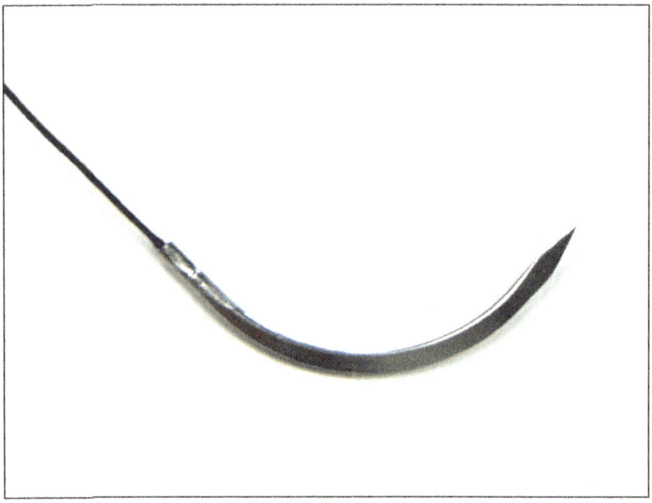

Now that we know the parts of a needle, we can look at how to pick different ones. This is based on a number of different attributes, and varies according to what you are trying to suture:

- **Needle length** –the choice of needle length is very much dictated by the thickness of the tissue you are suturing. So, if you are suturing an eyelid, this has very thin skin and a needle length of around 11mm could be appropriate. Trying to suture thick back skin with an 11mm needle would be difficult/impossible though, as the length of the needle can't reach the depth you need to produce a good closure. On the back therefore, you may need a needle of 26mm or more.

- **Needle shape** – needles come in various shapes, including straight, 'J' shaped and half-curved. The needle shown in the image above is the shape most commonly used in skin surgery, which is the curved needle.
- **Curve description** – the curve is described according to how much of a circle it describes. So a half-circle needle will have the shape of a half circle, a five-eighths (5/8) needle will look like 5/8 of a circle, and so on. The needle pictured is a 3/8 needle, which is my favourite for skin suturing.
- **Point** – the point can be various shapes including blunt, rounded and spatula-shaped, but in skin suturing I like the reverse-cutting point. This is a sharp-tipped needle, which is triangular when looked at in cross section, with the apex of the triangle pointing backwards. This helps the needle pass through the skin with the least trauma.

In summary, when suturing skin, my personal default is a 3/8 reverse cutting needle, with the length changing according to need. I tend to use an 11mm needle for eyelids, 16mm for other areas on the face, 19mm for the chest, abdomen or arms, and 26mm for the back or legs. This is by no means a fixed guide though, and skin thicknesses can change with age (thinner in very young or older patients) and you will no doubt find your own personal preferences in time.

Having chosen our needle, we need to decide on the thread we are going to use. Again, there is a wide range of different threads to choose from, but for skin suturing we can try to narrow things down to a few different choices:

- **Absorbable vs non-absorbable** – the non-absorbable suture threads are, as their name suggests, threads that don't dissolve. In skin suturing, these are generally used for suturing the outer layer of skin and are removed after a few days when the wound has healed. Absorbable sutures will dissolve, losing their strength as they do so. The time it takes for them to break down can vary, but generally the ones used for skin can range from taking just a few days to a few weeks or months to dissolve and lose their strength. Absorbable sutures are usually used in deeper layers of skin, keeping their strength for a few weeks and so allowing the scar strength to build and keep the wound closed (think of a wound closure on the front of the knee – every time the knee bends, the scar will come under pressure to pull open – a layer of deep absorbable sutures will hold the wound closed until the scar is strong enough). The top/outer layer of skin can also be closed with absorbable sutures, which take just a few days to lose their strength and fall out, but this does carry risks of inflammation, infection and 'suture mark' scarring. Generally, I use absorbable sutures for deep layers, when performing a continuous subcuticular closure (more on this later!), or very occasionally on scalps or small biopsy wounds.

- **Monofilament vs multifilament** – the monofilament threads are single smooth threads, whilst multifilament threads are numerous thin strands that are woven (braided) together. In skin suturing, the non-absorbable sutures tend to be monofilament whilst the absorbable ones can be monofilament or braided. Monofilament sutures glide more easily through tissue, but can cut through tissue if under too much tension; the braided sutures can be useful when closing deep tissue such as fat therefore,

as they grasp and tend to not cut through soft tissue as easily.
An exception to this is the silk suture, which is a braided non-absorbable suture. Silk is rarely (if ever) used in standard skin closures, but is commonly used in Plastic surgery to tie on a skin graft; more importantly for this book, silk sutures are also very handy as practice sutures as they are easy to handle and tie, are easy to see, and don't tear out of tissue (or practice pads) as easily as some other suture threads.

- **Specific composition** – the threads themselves can be made from different base material, which can alter the way they behave. Polypropylene for example, is commonly used as a non-absorbable suture but can be very springy (termed 'high memory') and not very pliable. Personally, I therefore prefer using a nylon thread to close top layers of skin, as I find this easier to handle. As always though, try different sutures to see what suits you best!

- **Thread strength** – the strength of a specific thread is proportional to the diameter (thickness) of thread. For skin suturing, you will come across the '-0' system, where the number before the '0' increases as the thread becomes thinner/weaker. So, if made from the same material, a 2/0 thread is thicker and stronger than a 5/0 thread. In microsurgery, an 11/0 suture may be used, which is extremely fine.
Ideally, you want to use the thinnest thread possible for the task in order to minimize trauma and scarring. As examples, I will tend to use a 5/0 or 6/0 thread on the face, and a 3/0 or 4/0 thread on the trunk or limbs.

Try not to worry too much about specific sutures at this point, it takes time to get used to the vast range of sutures available and you don't need to know them in order to practice. We do need to know more about the instruments though, and fortunately there aren't many you need to know about…..

Toothed forceps are shaped like tweezers, but have a noticeable feature – they have small interlocking teeth at their tips which are used to grasp tissue and maintain a firm hold. This is very useful when suturing skin, as you can hold a skin edge steady while passing a suture needle through it. Take care when using toothed forceps though, as the pointed teeth can easily cause trauma to tissue if the forceps are pinched too tightly. The forceps are usually held in a 'pen' or 'chopstick' grip, where they rest on the middle finger to allow the thumb and index finger to pinch the forceps arms. They are held in your non-dominant hand, so that your dominant hand can do the trickier work in suturing.

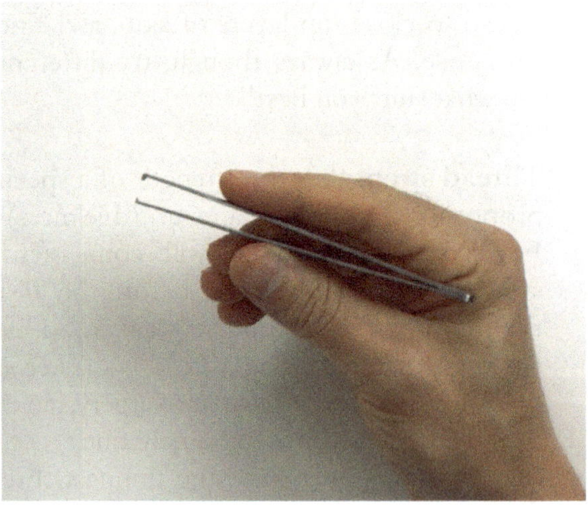

Needle holders (also called 'needle drivers', especially in the USA) are, as their name suggests, used to hold the needle. The needle is held just back from the tips of the holder jaws, and about a third of the way down from the swage.

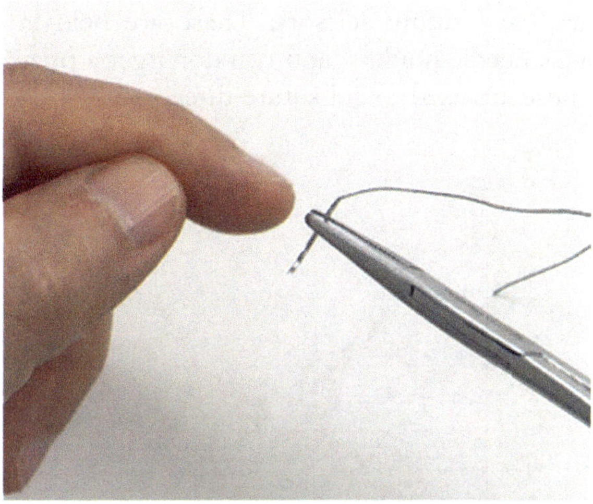

To hold the needle holders, place your thumb pulp in one of the handles, and the pulp of your ring finger into the other. Your index finger should then rest on the arms near the hinge, and your middle finger can rest on the side of the holders. This may feel a little strange at first but will soon become more natural.

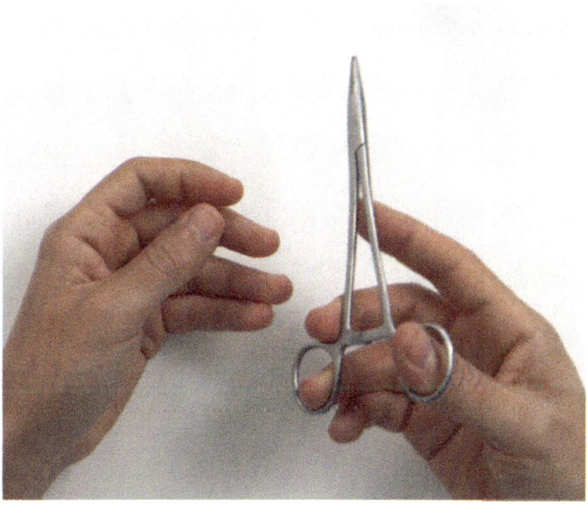

Finally, we have suture scissors. These are held in exactly the same way as needle holders, and you don't get a prize for figuring out that these are used to cut suture threads!

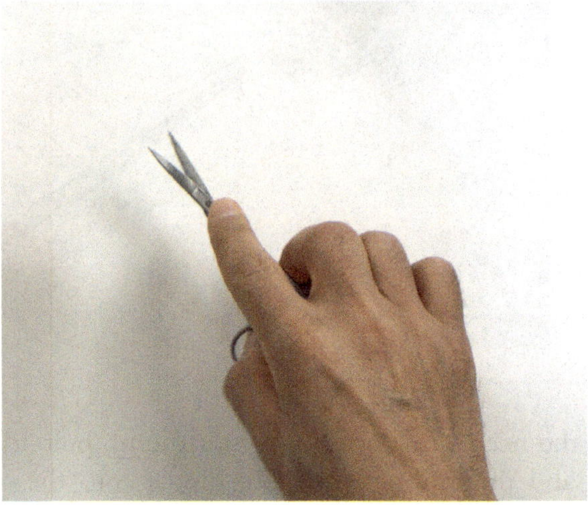

We're now ready to start developing our practical skills and learn to suture.......

3 PASSING THE NEEDLE

When you push a needle through the skin, we call this 'passing' the needle. This skill is a foundation of suturing, and unfortunately is commonly performed badly, which is why I want to spend a whole chapter on this.

A key movement in passing the needle actually comes from your wrist and forearm, whereby pronation and supination of your hand helps pass the needle with the least trauma to the skin. **Pronation** is where your hand rotates to face palm-downwards. When your hand turns to be palm up, this is **supination** (think 'holding a bowl of *soup* needs *sup*ination'). We can practice this movement on the edge of a suture pad. First, load your needle in the needle holder, by holding the needle just down from (proximal to) the tips of the jaws. The needle should be held approximately one-third down from the swage.

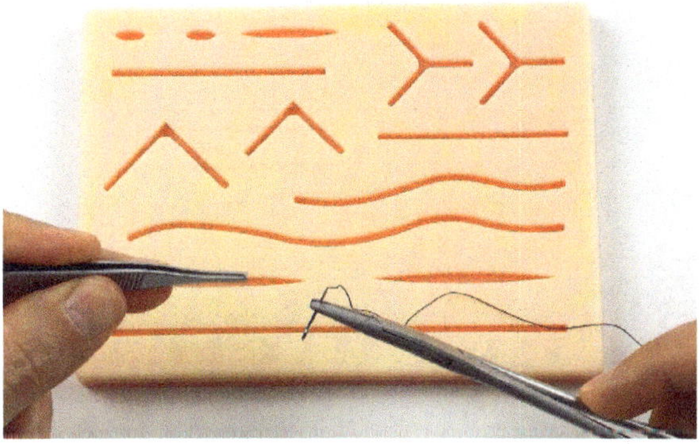

Slightly pronate your hand, and you will see that this rotates the needle. You are aiming to be able to enter the pad at 90 degrees to the surface.

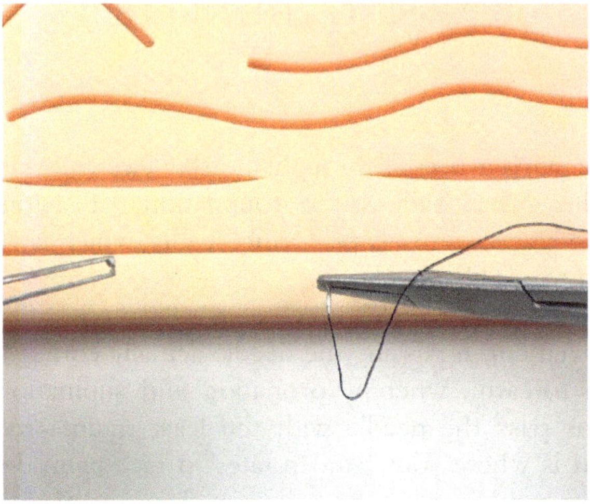

Start to push the needle into the pad, about 3-4mm from the edge. You can use your toothed forceps to gently stabilize the pad while you do this, but try to not grasp it too tightly.

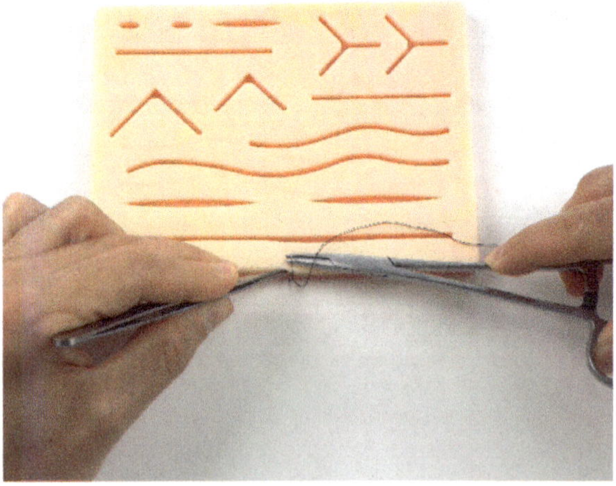

Keep pushing the needle through, using a combination of gentle pushing and supination (turning your hand clockwise) as you do so. This should aim to allow the needle to travel through the skin by following the curved shape of the needle. Release the needle holders and grasp the needle that has appeared from the deeper aspect of the pad, around 3-4mm from the surface.

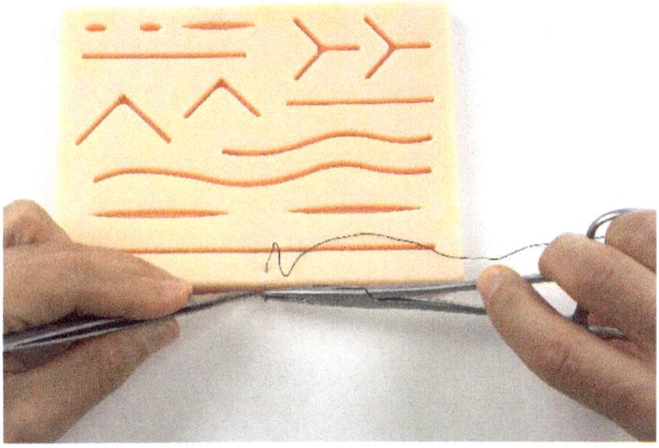

You can now use a combination of supination and gentle pulling to pull the needle free. Again, allow the needle to follow its curve, don't just pull the needle straight out. Keep pulling until the thread has been fully pulled out.

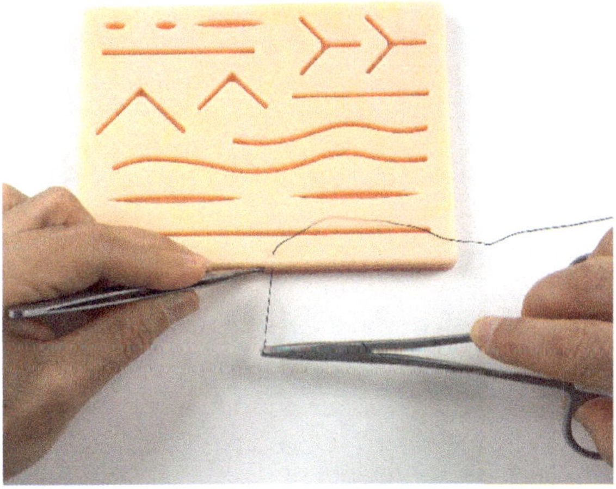

Alternatively, if you are using a long thread, pull the thread towards you by flexing your arm at the elbow. To then remove the rest of the thread from the pad, use your 'spare' hand (the one with the forceps) to pull it free. In real life, the 'forceps hand' is often used in this way to assist.

Keep repeating this exercise until you feel confident, then it's time to move on!

4 THE INSTRUMENT TIE

Now that we have seen how to pass a needle, we can turn to the next crucial skill in suturing – the instrument tie. This is where a knot is tied in the suture thread, using both your needle holders and your hands.

We start with a needle having been passed through the pad edge, and the thread pulled until around an inch (25mm) is left loose.

Now put your toothed forceps down, or hold them in your palm, while you grasp the long end of the thread (the end with the needle attached).
Place the needle holders on top of the thread, then wrap the thread twice around the arms of the holders.

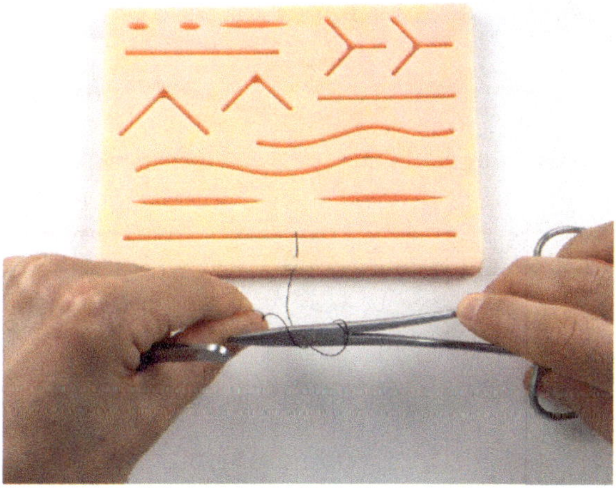

Now grasp the short end of the thread with the tips of the needle holders.

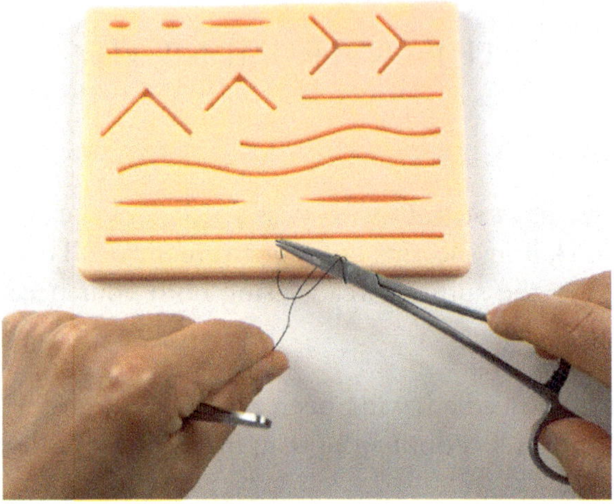

Pull the short thread through and towards you, while you push the long end away from you. Snug this down to the pad. By moving your hands in these directions, the tie should be neat and not twisted, and look like the picture below.

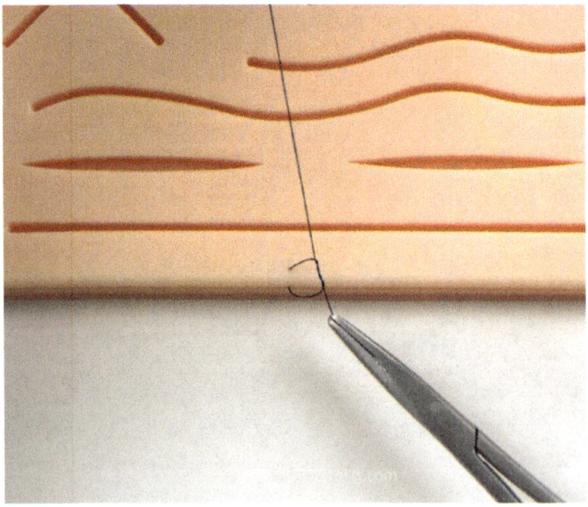

Then take the long thread over the holders and wrap it around them once.

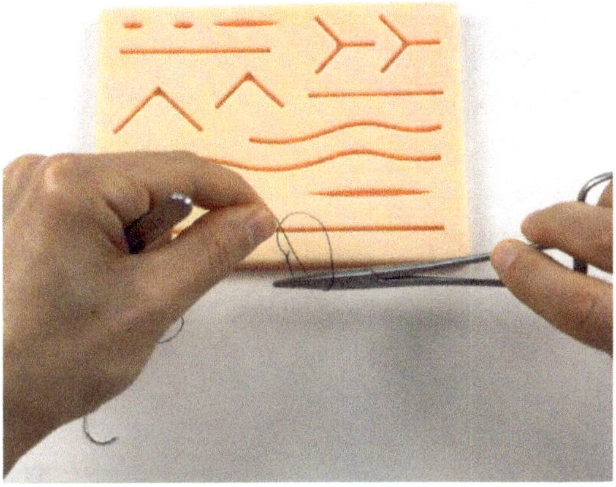

Grasp the short end of the thread with the tips of the needle holders and push it away from you while pulling the long thread towards you. Snug the throw down until it forms a knot. Again, if you have moved your hands correctly, the throw will be neat and not twisted, as shown below.

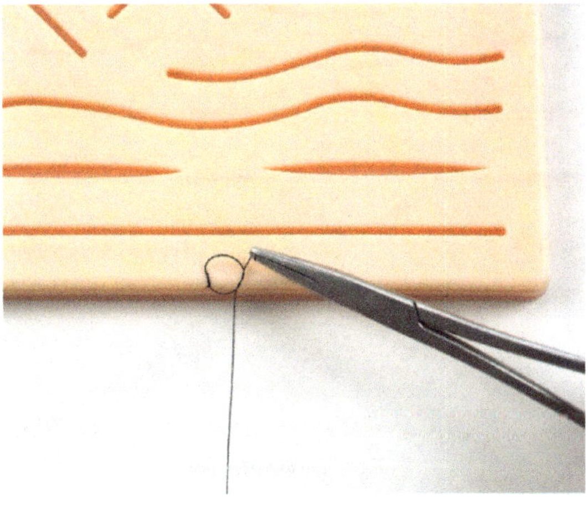

We need one more throw to secure the knot. Place the holders over the thread, and wrap the thread around once.

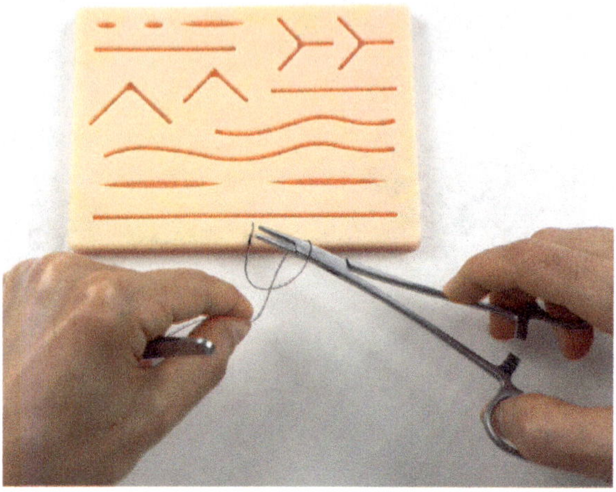

Grasp the short end of the thread, and pull it towards you while pushing the long thread away from you, forming a neat throw.

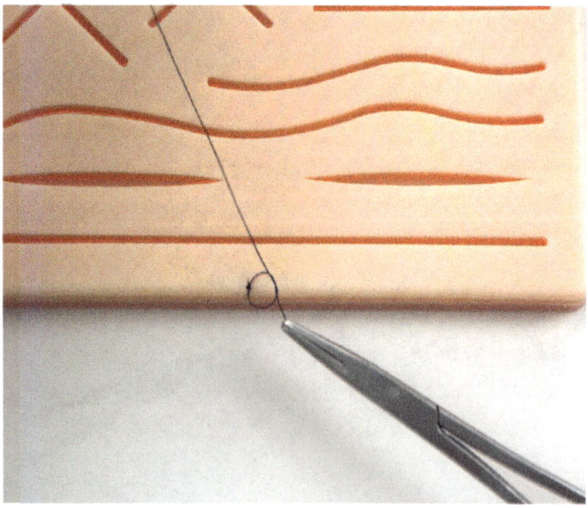

Snug this throw down to secure your knot. This can now be cut with your scissors, leaving 'tails' of around 1cm.

Top tips:

- When grasping the thread with your needle holders, try to not engage the locking ratchet at the handle. I say this because if you do, then you need to unlock it to then let go of the thread. This can quickly lead to tired and sore hands, and will add time and inefficiency to your suturing. Instead, try to grasp the thread firmly enough to allow a tie but not so tight as to engage the ratchet lock.
- Take care to follow the correct order of hands crossing over. Your loops should be nice and neatly 'squared' as shown in the pictures. If you have your hands travelling in the wrong direction then you will see your loops are twisted, leading to knots that are prone to loosening and failing.
- Don't ever grasp the long part of the thread with your needle holders. The jaws of the holders are rough and can abrade the suture, leading to it breaking. In real life this could be a crucial suture that breaks!

Congratulations, you're now well on your way and it's time to start to suture a wound!

5 INTERRUPTED SUTURES

Having practiced the separate components, we are now ready to move on and start suturing. We're starting with the most basic, and most often used, suture – the interrupted suture (don't forget, 'suture' is also another word for 'stitch'). It is called 'interrupted' because the thread is interrupted, or cut, between each suture.

We are going to start by passing our needle through one side of the wound on a suture pad. Our needle is loaded, holding it near the tips of the holders and about one-third down from the swage. Our toothed forceps are in the other hand.

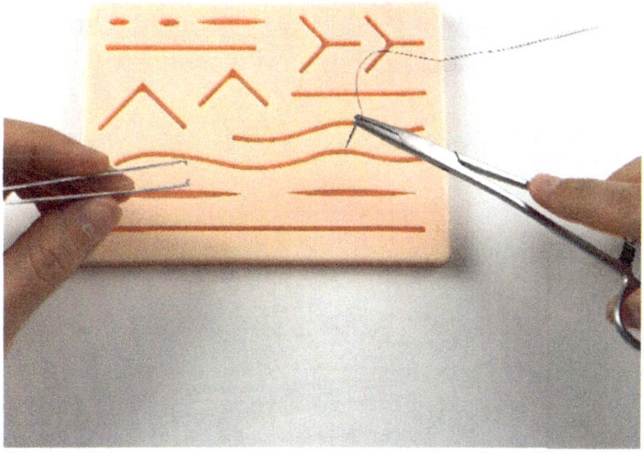

As you practiced before, pronate your hand so that the needle point can enter the surface at 90 degrees, about 3-4mm from the wound edge (note the right hand is pronated in the image below).

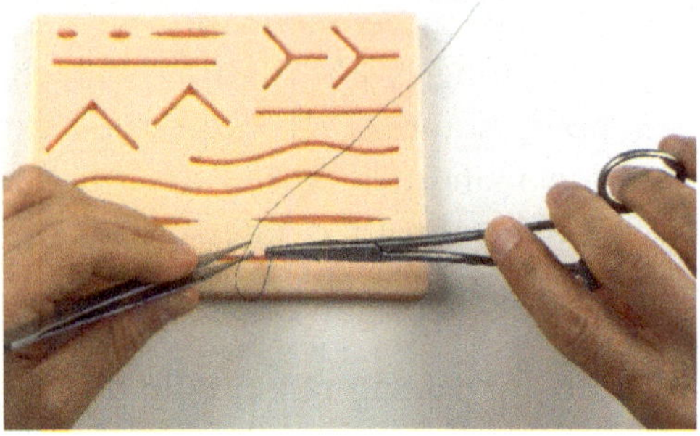

Through pushing and supination, make the needle point appear in the wound, around 3-4mm from the surface. You can use the toothed forceps to push against the skin and provide counter-pressure while you pass the needle; you can also hold the edge of the skin with the forceps, but if you do so then try to not hold the skin too tightly or you could crush it (in real life, this can lead to worse scarring, delayed healing and infection).

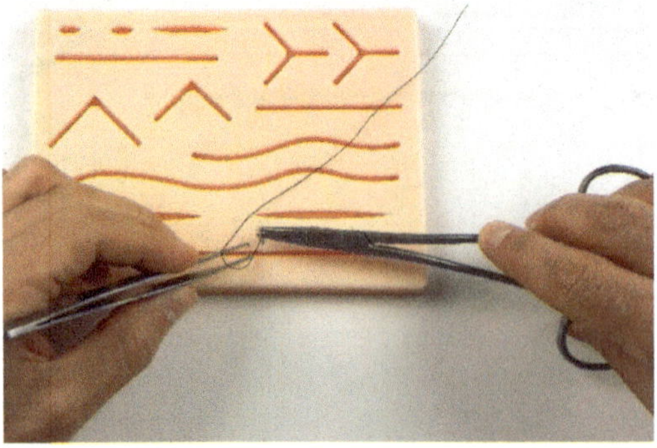

Release the needle holders, grasp the distal part of the needle (the part showing through in the wound), and supinate your hand while pulling the needle through, allowing the needle to follow its curve.

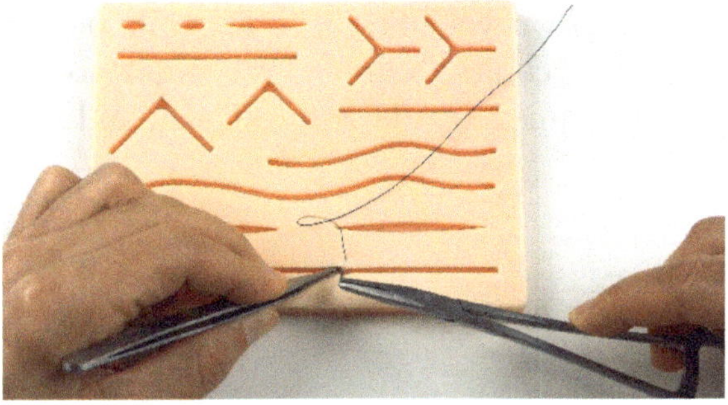

We can now pass the needle through the opposite wound edge. Push the needle point into the deep aspect of the other side, about 3-4mm deep and directly opposite to where it has just been pulled free. Push the needle, allowing it to follow its curve by supinating your hand, so that the tip appears at the surface around 3-4mm from the wound edge. You can use your toothed forceps to help by applying counter-pressure to the wound surface as the tip appears, or gently grasp the wound edge.

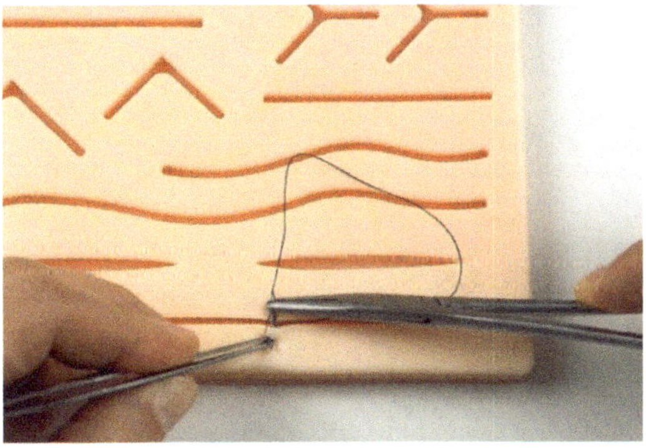

Now release the needle holders, grasp the needle near the tip, and pull it out whilst supinating your hand.

We're now ready to tie our suture, using the 'instrument tie' technique described earlier.

When tightening down your first throw, gently tighten until the wound edges just come together. We want to avoid over-tightening, as the thread can dig into the skin and lead to worse scarring.

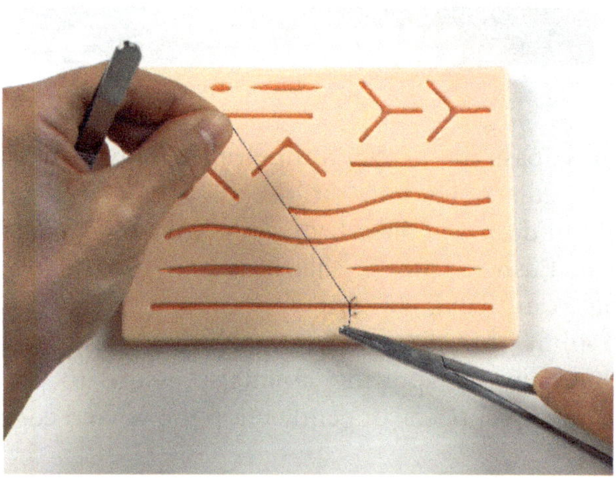

You can now perform the next two steps of the instrument tie, snugging your throws down to form a neat knot. Cut your thread to leave 'tails' of about 10mm.

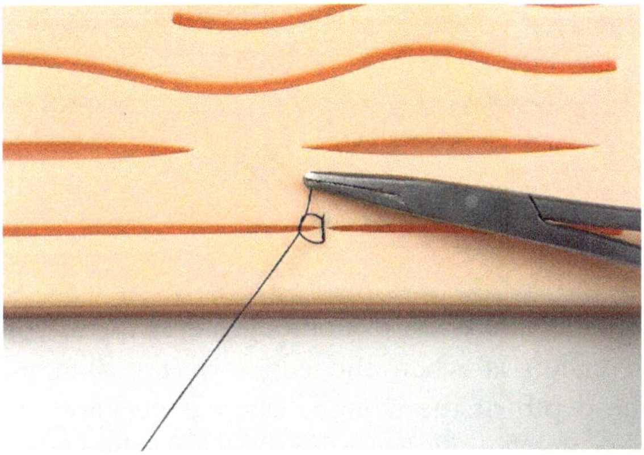

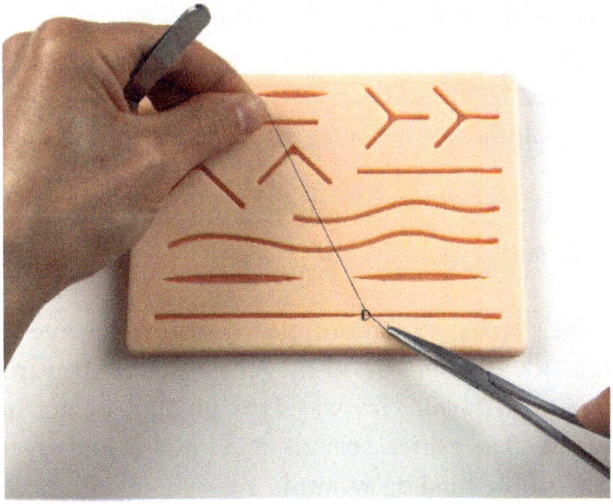

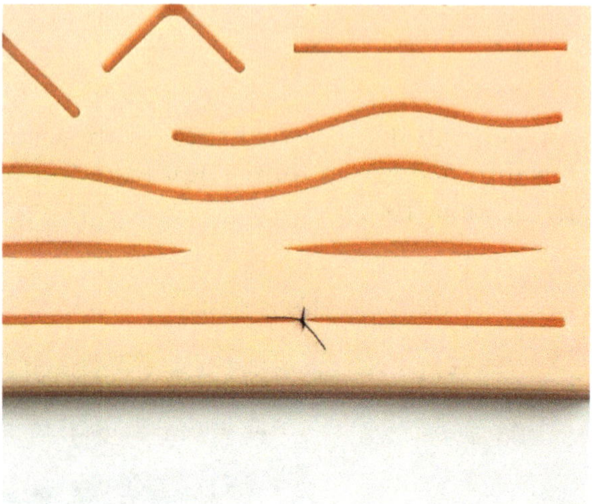

Hopefully, you will see the wound edges everting as you close the wound; inversion is when the edges of the skin point down towards the depth of the wound, whereas eversion is where the edges pucker up slightly. Eversion allows for better skin healing, and so better scarring (although we do occasionally aim for inversion when reconstructing specific 'indented' areas such as the nose/cheek junction). Don't worry if you don't see eversion to start with; with practice and by taking care to follow these steps, you should hopefully start to achieve this.

Repeat this across the wound, leaving around 8-10mm gaps between each suture placement.

Once you are getting confident, see if you can leave your knots on the same side of the wound by gently pulling towards yourself as you snug down your throws. This gives a neater appearance and can result in a better scar as it avoids knots overlying and interfering with the healing wound.

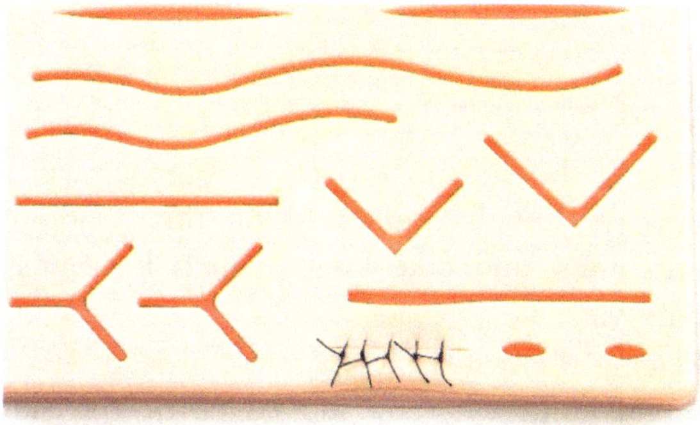

Advantages:

- This is the 'workhorse' suture, which can be used in most scenarios when suturing skin.
- You can accurately approximate skin edges, useful when joining important landmarks, complex shaped wounds or tattooed skin.
- It is also useful for making fine adjustments as you close the wound, for example when the two wound edges are not the same length.
- The gaps between the sutures allows for a degree of wound swelling and so may lead to better healing.
- If a single suture fails, the rest of the wound will remain closed as the other sutures are still intact.

Disadvantages:

- It can take a long time to close long or multiple wounds.
- Removing a large number of individual sutures can be time consuming.

Top tips:

- Placing the sutures too close together will take more time, potentially reduce blood flow leading to worse outcomes, and take longer when it comes to suture removal.
- Placing them too far apart could lead to 'gapping' of the wound, whereby the edges of the skin are not closely approximated. This can lead to delayed healing and worse scarring.
- Pronating and supinating your hand when placing the needle is crucial to it entering and travelling through the skin in the correct pathway, leading to eversion (pouting) of the wound edges. Without eversion, there is more risk of poorer healing and cosmesis.

6 CRUCIATE SUTURE

The cruciate suture is similar to the interrupted suture and can be useful for long straight wounds.

We start by passing the needle through both sides of the wound in the same manner as for an interrupted suture. As you become more confident, you can try passing through both edges at the same time as shown in the image below.

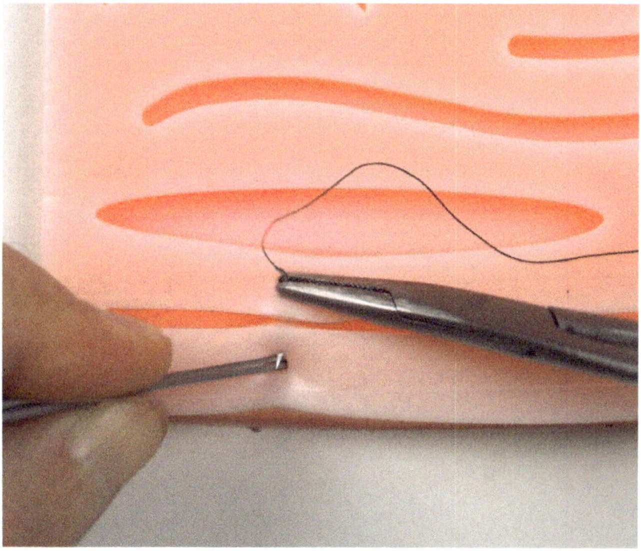

Rather than tying a knot at this point, we repeat the same movement, approximately 5mm along the wound.

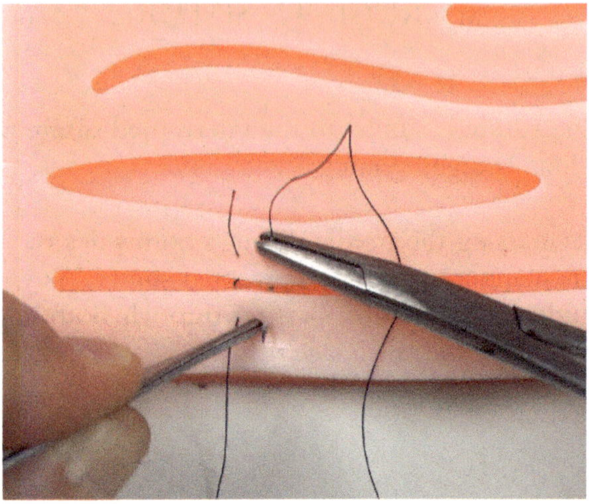

Having performed two passes, the suture is now ready to tie off.

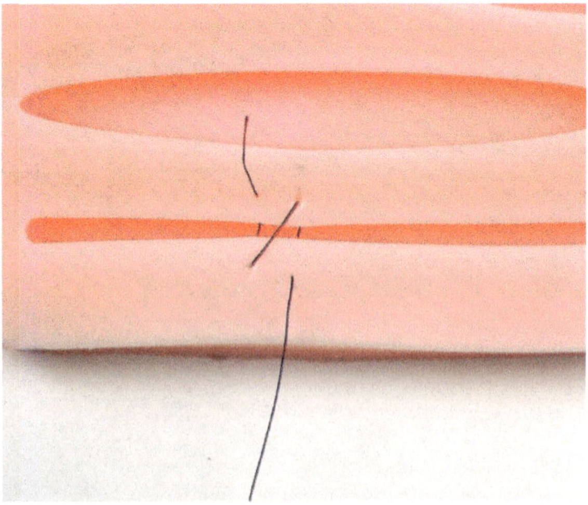

Perform an instrument tie, aiming to place the knot on one side of the wound.

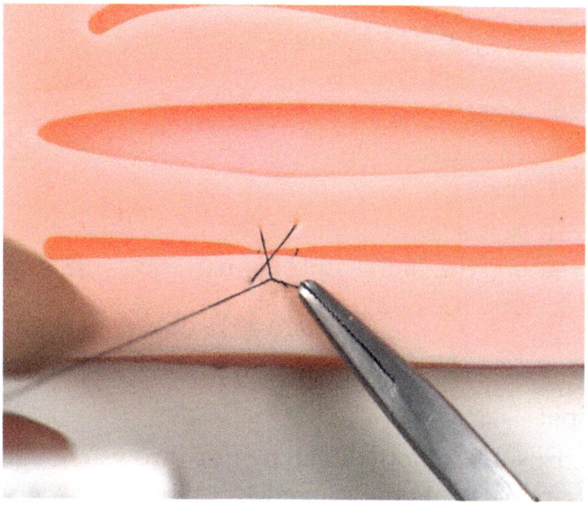

Cut the thread, leaving short 'tails'. You can now repeat the suture until the wound is closed.

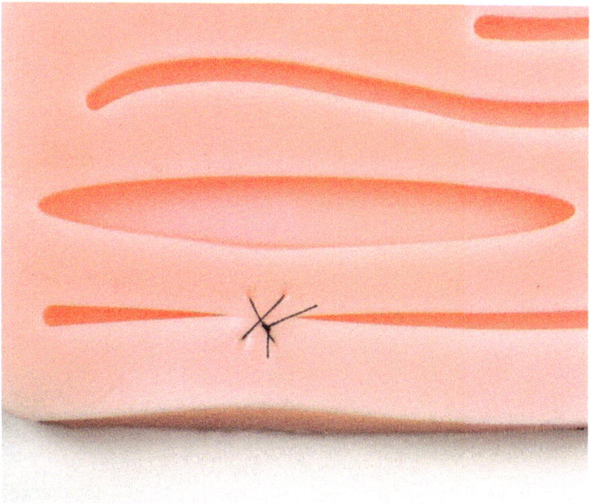

Advantages:

- This is similar to the interrupted suture but can shorten the time it takes to close long wounds.
- It is an easily mastered suture.

Disadvantages:

- It can easily be over-tightened, leading to worse scarring.
- It is not as accurate and precise as the interrupted suture for lining up landmarks or fine areas such as around the eyelid.

Top tips:

- Ensure you only tighten your throws enough to gently approximate the skin edges.
- Don't space the two passes too far apart as this can cause 'bunching' of the skin and a less neat closure.
- Placing the passes too close together leads to more suture material and trauma to the wound with little advantage over a simple interrupted suture.

7 CONTINUOUS SUTURE

The continuous suture is a useful technique for closing wounds quickly, for example when a patient is extremely unwell so would be at risk with a lengthy general anaesthetic. The continuous suture can easily be over-tightened though, leading to poorer scarring, so care must be taken.

We start by performing an interrupted suture, but this time don't cut the main thread. Instead, reload the needle in the holders.

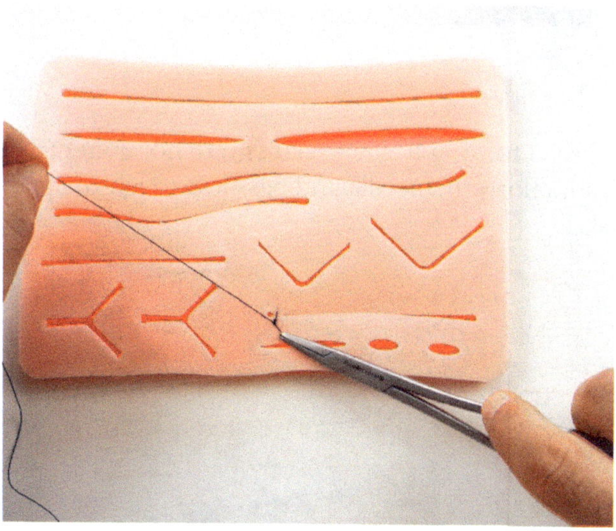

Approximately 6-8mm from this suture, perform the motions for another interrupted suture by passing the needle through both sides of the wound.

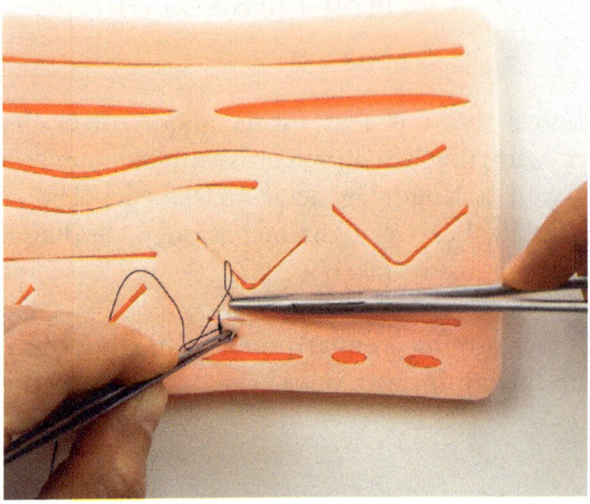

Pull the thread to snug it down, but you're not going to tie a knot yet. Instead, reload the needle and pass it through the pad again.

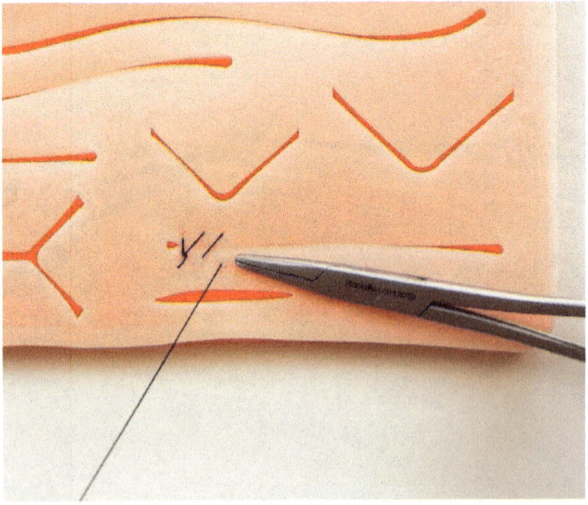

Keep repeating this until the wound is closed. When you reach the end , leave the last thread loose.

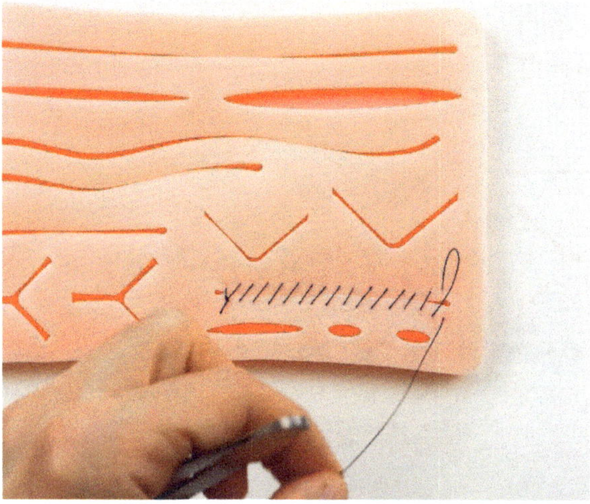

We can now tie our knot. This is in the same way as a standard instrument tie, but whereas we normally grasp the short end of the thread after throwing the thread around the holders, we are instead going to grasp the loop to perform our knots.

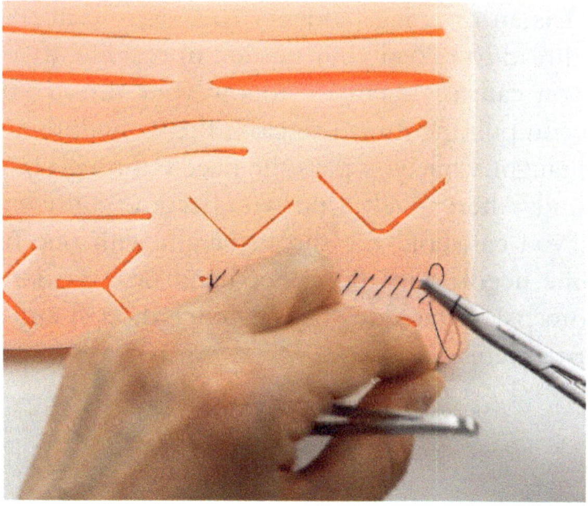

Once you have performed your instrument tie, you can cut your threads to leave 'tails' of around 1cm.

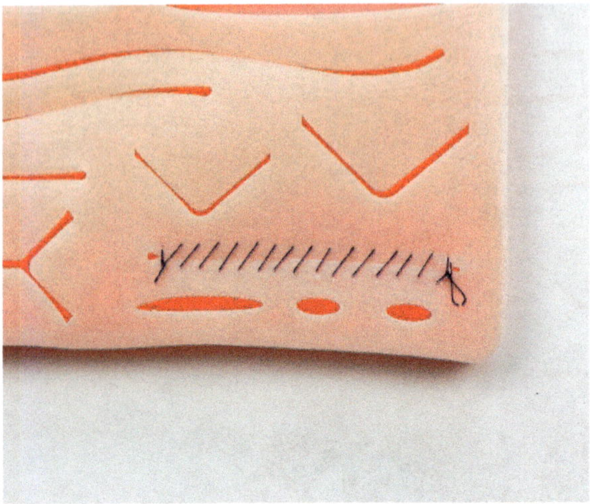

As explained earlier, it is easy to over-tighten this suture, leading to worse scarring. To try and avoid this, make sure you pull on the thread gently to only just close the wound after each time you pass the needle through. You'll find though that this suture technique has an irritating tendency to loosen itself once you let go of the thread to reload your needle. In real life, if you have an assistant, you can ask them to 'follow your thread'; this means that when you pull the thread to close the wound, they then hold the thread taught while you pass the needle through the next part of the wound. Alternatively, once you become confident with the technique, you can hold the thread taught with one hand while you pass the needle with the other hand (ie, you don't use the toothed forceps) – this does take practice though and can easily cause over-tightening.

Advantages:

- A great suture technique for rapid closure of long or multiple wounds. Such scenarios could include a very unwell patient that can only have a short general anaesthetic or a clinically unstable patient in A&E/ER.

Disadvantages:

- This suture is prone to over-tightening, so can lead to worse scarring.
- Failure (breakage) of any part of the suture can lead to the entire suture line loosening and the wound dehiscing (splitting open).
- It can be difficult to accurately approximate aesthetic landmarks.

Top tips:

- Take note of the spacing between passes; placing the sutures too close together will take more time, potentially reduce blood flow leading to worse outcomes, and take longer when it comes to suture removal. Placing them too far apart could lead to 'gapping' of the wound, whereby the edges of the skin are not closely approximated. This can lead to delayed healing and worse scarring. Trying to pull the thread tighter to compensate for this leads to even worse results.
- Use your forceps hand, or an assistant, to hold the thread taught while you place your next pass. Don't pull too hard as this will over-tighten the thread. Just pull enough to prevent your previous throws from loosening.
- For very long wounds, you can break the suture length up. Rather than closing the wound in one long section,

you can close it with 3,4 or more sections of continuous suture. This means you close the wound in less time than if interrupted sutures were used, whilst allowing for more accurate approximation of the skin and giving less chance of cumulative over-tightening of throws. In addition, failure of part of a thread means only a section of the wound may dehisce, rather than the entire wound.

8 CONTINUOUS LOCKED SUTURE

This can be a useful extension of the continuous suture; if your continuous suture keeps loosening because you don't have an assistant or because the wound is under tension, then you can lock each pass to avoid this loosening. You may also find that locking each pass can help you better achieve wound eversion.

We start in the same way as a standard continuous suture, by performing an interrupted suture but keeping the thread attached. Then pass your needle through the wound edges, but when you see the needle tip appear, don't pull it out just yet; first, make sure the loop of loose thread is lying below the needle tip.

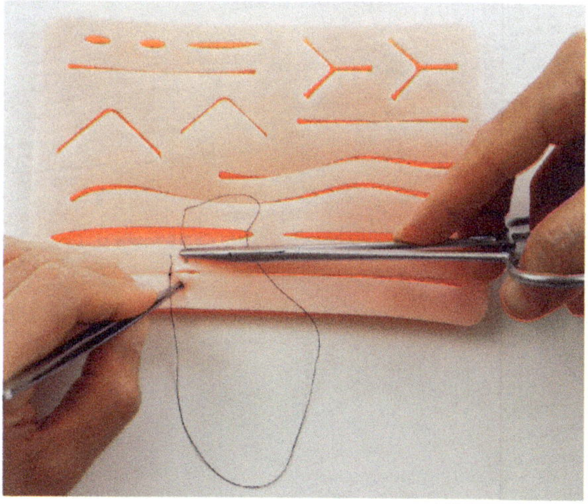

Then pull the needle out so that it passes through the loop. Pull on the thread so that the wound starts to close.

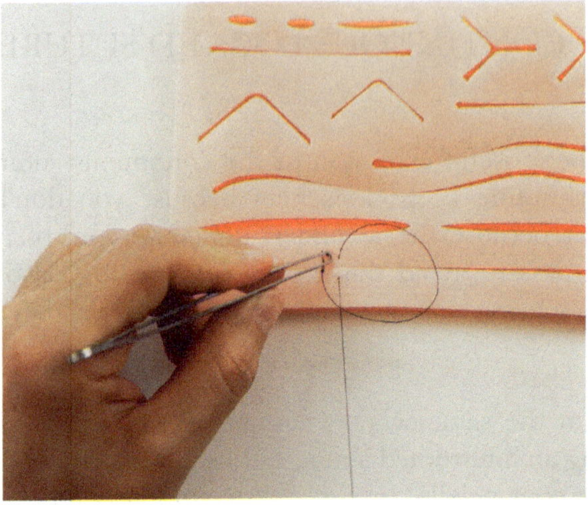

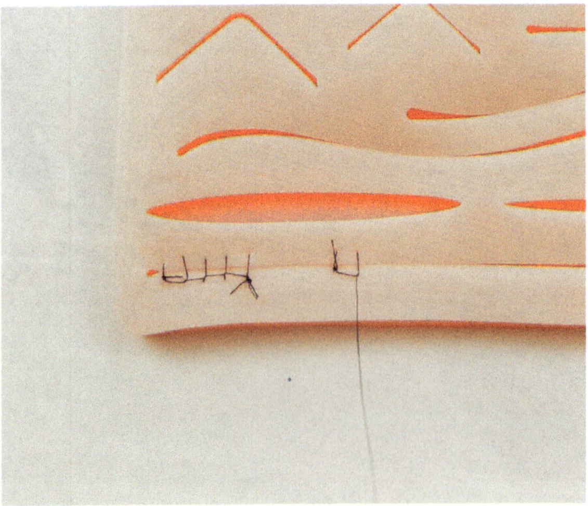

Now repeat – pass the needle as if you were performing a continuous suture, but again make sure the loose thread is below the needle when it is pulled free from the wound, making the needle pass through the loop each time.

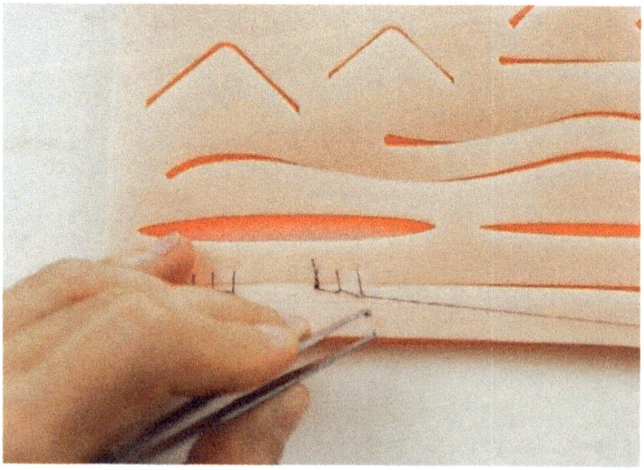

Each time you tighten the thread, do so by pulling towards you. This will make the 'locks' lie on one side of the wound. If needed you can use your 'forceps hand' to hold the thread taught and prevent it loosening, or ask an assistant to do this if one is available.

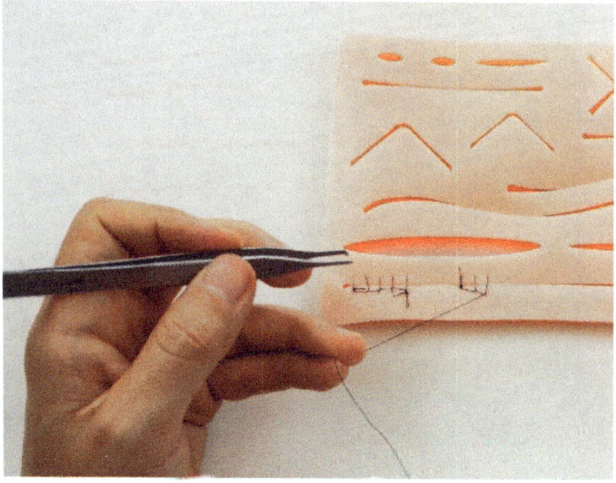

Keep progressing until the wound is closed. The suturing is again ended by using a loop to tie your knot.

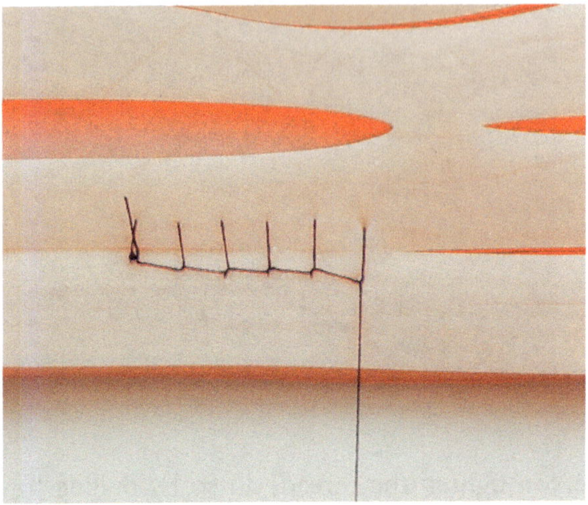

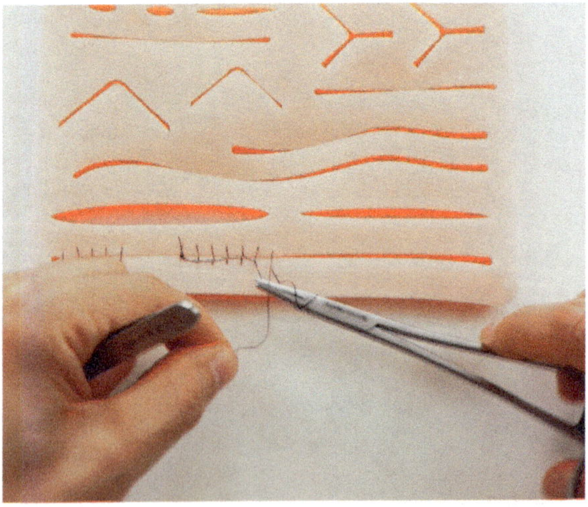

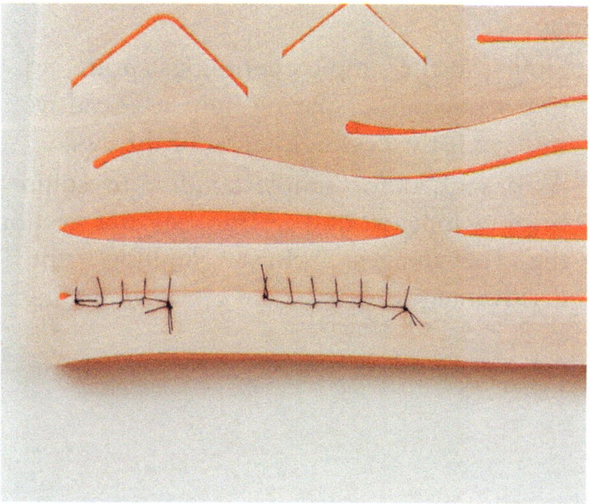

As with the continuous suture, you need to take care to not over-tighten your throws as this can lead to worse scarring.

Advantages:

- Similar to the simple continuous suture, this technique is useful for rapid closure of long wounds.
- Locking the throws can allow for more controlled tension in the closure as compared to the standard continuous suture.
- The locks can help you evert the wound edges.

Disadvantages:

- Due to the locks, removing the sutures can be more fiddly and take longer than a simple continuous suture.
- If part of it breaks, then the locks may help prevent instant loosening of the suture but ultimately the integrity of the entire closure is lost.

Top tips:

- Similar to the simple continuous suture, it is important to get the suture spacing right to avoid wound gaping or need for excess tightening of throws.
- As described for simple continuous sutures, you can break a long wound up into shorter sections to gain the advantages whilst limiting the potential disadvantages.

We hope you're enjoying this book and learning lots!
If you'd like to learn more about suturing, performing minor procedures and surgery tips & tricks, head to Surgeryskills.com and sign up to one of our courses……..

Use these codes for 20% off these courses:
Suturing skills – 'Suture20'
Minor procedures – 'Procedure20'

And as a special book offer, get our 'Introduction to surgery' course absolutely free. No catch, just a big thank you for reading this book!
Use code 'IntroFree' when signing up to the course to get it for free
(RRP £59).

All courses are pre-filmed so you can take them at home and in your own time. And you get a certificate for your CV/portfolio!

(Unfortunately, we can only continue these offers while funding allows, so may end at any time)

9 HORIZONTAL MATTRESS SUTURE

Mattress sutures are a very handy technique if you're having difficulty achieving wound eversion (making the edges of the wound 'pucker up'). This is especially the case when suturing the skin of palms or soles, as the skin in these areas has an annoying tendency to invert when being closed.

We start by passing the needle through both sides of the wound, as if we were performing an interrupted suture.

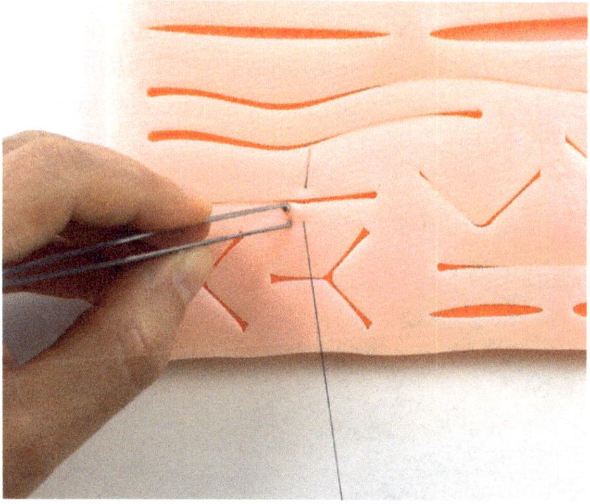

We're now going to reverse the needle. This involves having the needle in the holders so that it is pointing backwards.

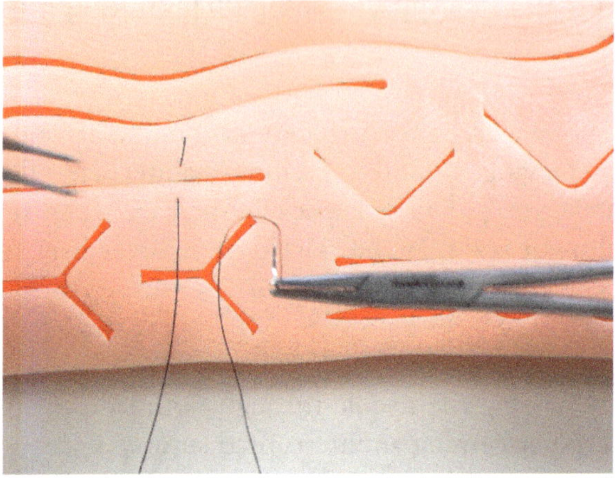

The needle is now placed approximately 5mm along from its last exit point, ensuring the needle enters at 90 degrees to the skin. You will need to supinate your hand (rotate clockwise) so that the needle can enter at the correct angle.

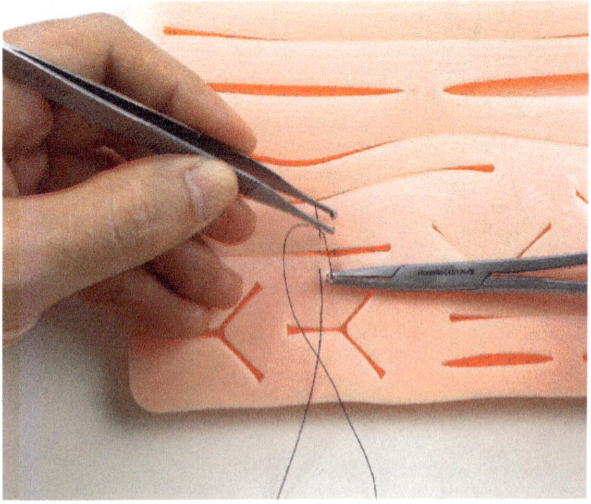

Pass the needle through both sides of the wound, so that it exits 5mm from your starting point.

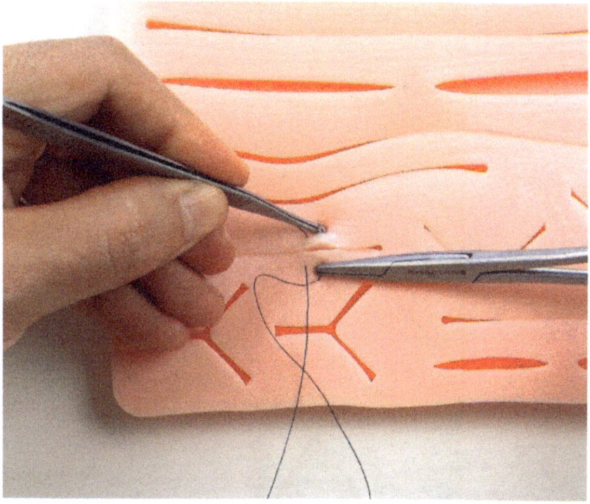

Pull the threads so that the wound closes. You should hopefully see that the wound edges are forced into eversion (puckering up).

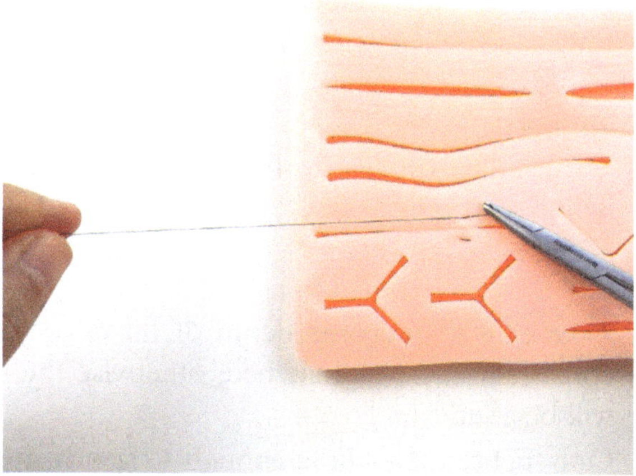

Perform an instrument tie to form a neat knot. Repeat the suture along the wound edges until it is closed.

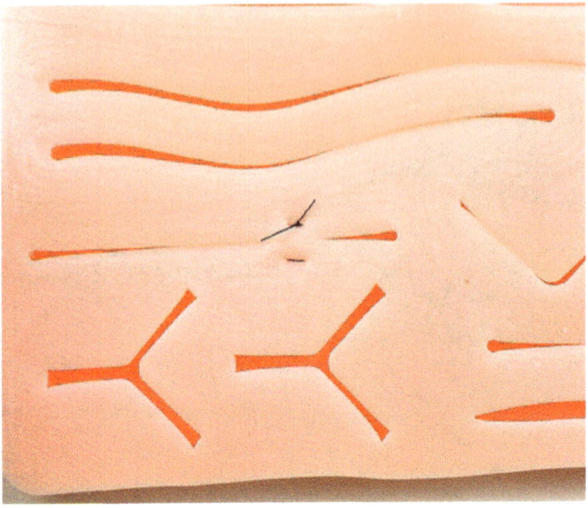

Advantages:

- This is a useful technique for skin closures that are prone to inversion, such as the palms or soles.
- As the suture 'grasps' tissue, it is also helpful when closing wounds under tension or if skin is a little fragile.

Disadvantages:

- This suture can easily be over-tightened, leading to worse scarring.

Top tips:

- Take care to keep the depth of travel of your needle consistent and well-matched, otherwise the skin edges will be at uneven levels.
- Only tighten the knots enough to gently approximate the skin edges and slightly evert the edges.

10 VERTICAL MATTRESS SUTURE

The vertical mattress suture is similarly used to help evert wound edges in areas that are prone to inversion.

Start by passing the needle through both sides of the wound, but this time keep the entry and exit points a little further away from the skin edges – start/exit around 6-8mm from the edges (we are performing it next to a horizontal mattress suture, so you can compare how they look). Aim for the deep dermis with this first pass, around 4-5mm from the surface.

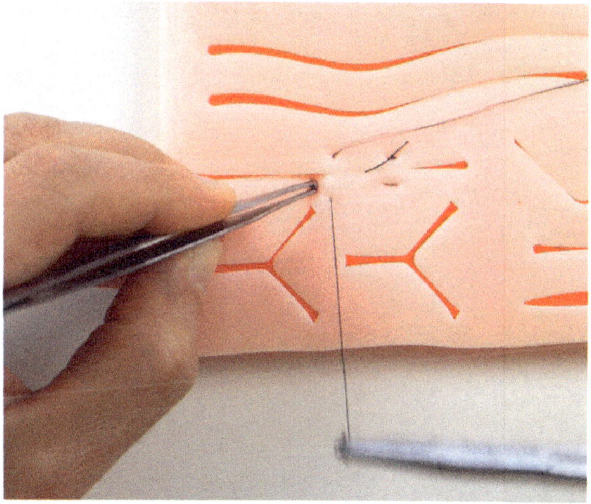

Now reverse your needle and pass it back through both edges, but this time around 3mm from the edges and 2-3mm from the surface. Unlike the horizontal mattress suture, we are going to perform this in line with our first pass.

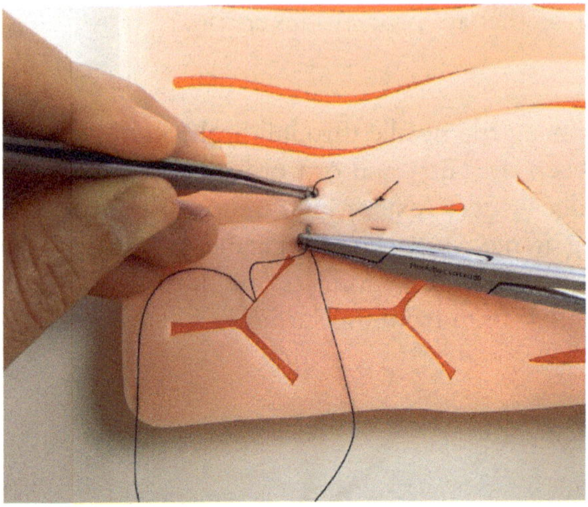

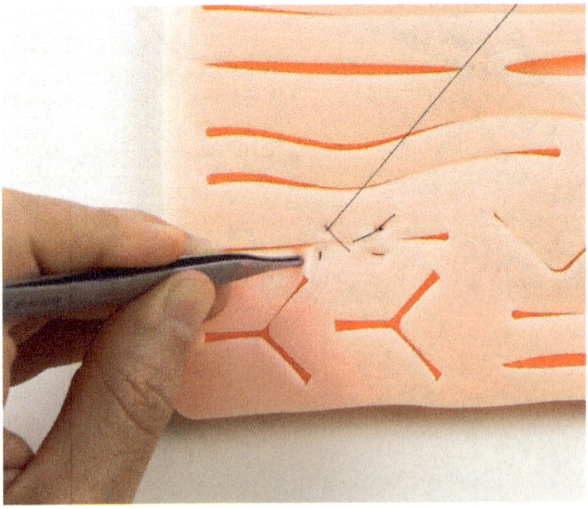

An instrument tie can now be performed to form a neat knot and force the wound edges into eversion. Repeat the process until your wound has been closed.

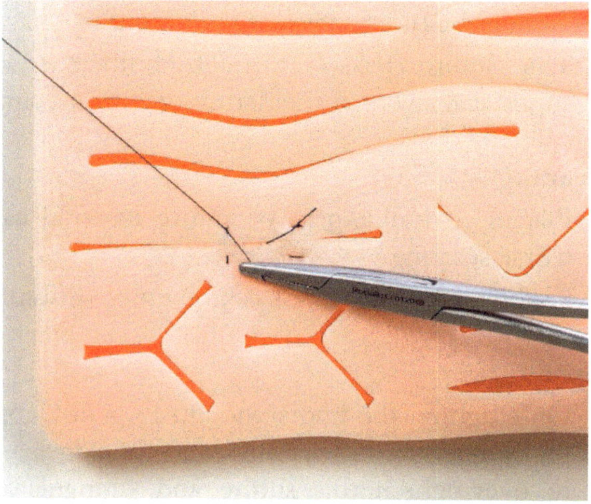

In the image below, you can see the difference between horizontal and vertical mattress sutures – the horizontal suture lies in a horizontal plane, whilst the vertical mattress suture (not surprisingly) lies in a vertical fashion.

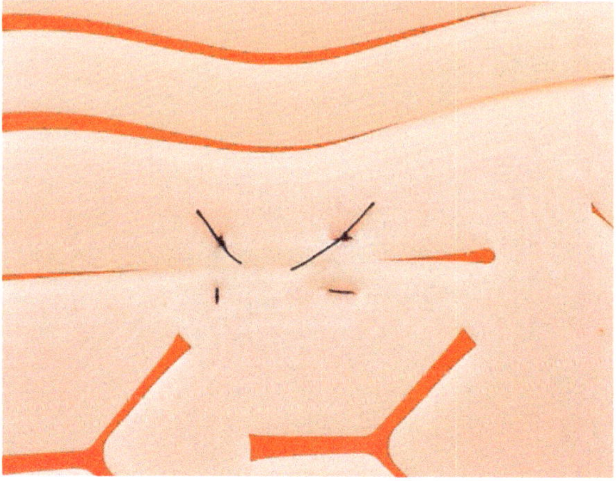

Advantages:

- Like the horizontal mattress, this is a useful technique for skin closures that are prone to inversion, and in fact can be more effective in doing this.
- The suture passes through both the deep and superficial layers of the dermis, giving a secure closure.

Disadvantages:

- Placing a double-pass of suture material can lead to worse scarring.
- Closing lengthy wounds can be time-consuming.

Top tips:

- Only tighten the knots enough to gently approximate the skin edges and slightly evert the edges as it is easy to over-tighten this suture and strangulate the skin edges.

11 SUBCUTICULAR INTERRUPTED SUTURE

This is a really important technique to learn as it brings wound edges closer together in readiness for the surface skin closure. This means that the skin closure is under less tension, producing better scars, and gives the wound more strength while it heals.

Start by using your toothed forceps to gently hold the skin edge closest to you. Pull the edge towards you so that you can see the deep aspect (in real life, the dermis). Now place your needle tip in the deep aspect and enter the wound edge, gently pushing the needle forwards until it exits around 1-2 mm from the skin surface. You will need to supinate your hand to allow the needle to smoothly travel along its curvature.

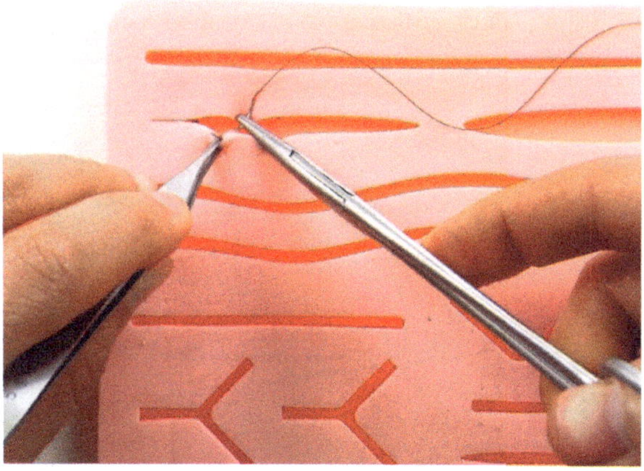

Reload the needle and hold the opposite wound edge with your forceps. The needle point now enters the wound edge directly opposite to where it has just exited. The needle point should be entering at 90 degrees, so you will need to pronate your hand to allow for this.

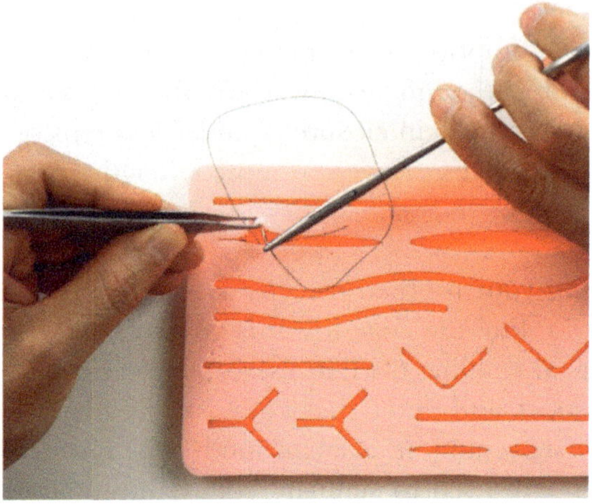

Gently push the needle through so that the point emerges from the wound edge, deep in the wound and directly opposite to where you first started.

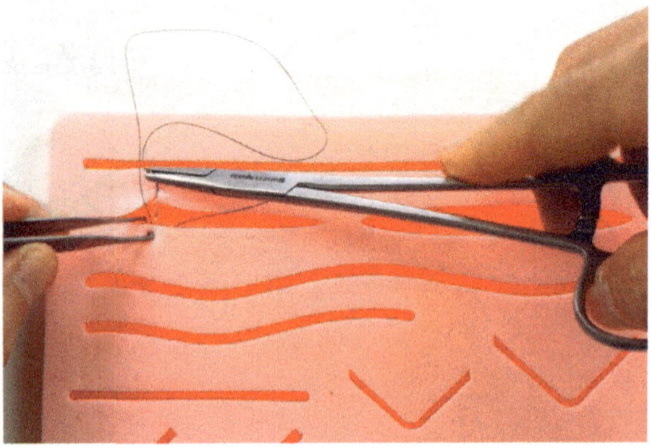

You can now perform your instrument tie. This is going to be a little trickier than usual as it is in the depth of the wound. You will see that your knot is now in the deep part of the wound, not near the surface. This is important in real life, as otherwise a knot near the surface could cause irritation and even extrude from the surface.

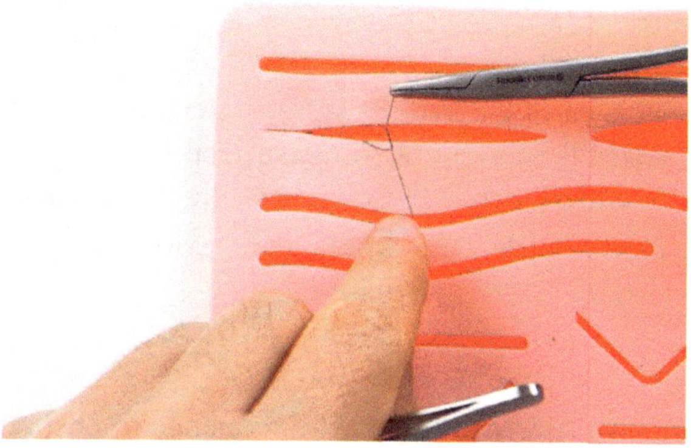

Cut the thread close to the knot so that the 'tails' are not too long. If they are too long, they could poke up through the wound and cause irritation. You will see that your wound edges are approximated (closed together) in an 'invisible' way.

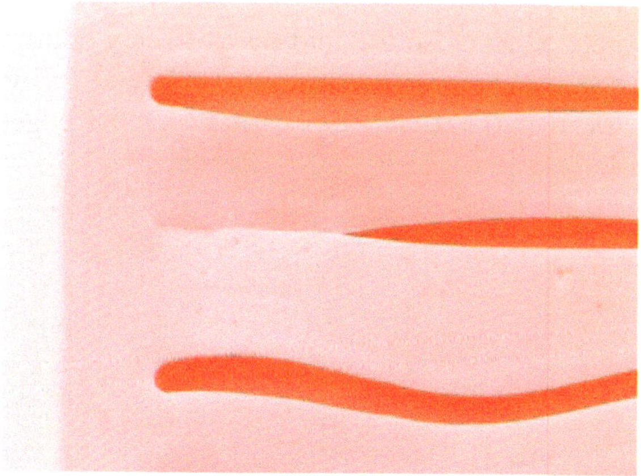

Advantages:

- This technique helps close the deep layer of wounds, allowing the skin surface to then be closed under minimal tension and lead to better scarring.
- Closing the deep layer adds strength to the wound during healing, giving less chance of wound dehiscence or scar stretching/widening.

Disadvantages:

- This can be a tricky suture to perform, especially if the space is quite tight (the last deep suture, when the rest of the wound is closed, is usually the trickiest!).
- Occasionally the knots can work their way to the surface, causing irritation.

Top tips:

- Make sure you follow the sequence to ensure the knots lie in the deep aspect of the wound when tied.
- Using a clear suture means that if you inadvertently place the suture too close to the surface, it won't be visible through the skin.
- Start at either end of the wound and work towards the middle with each successive suture. This gradually brings the edges together and reduces the tension needed to close the mid-part of the wound; starting at the mid-point when the wound is at its widest may mean it is difficult to neatly bring the edges together and tie a neat knot under tension.

12 SUBCUTICULAR CONTINUOUS SUTURE

I'm not going to lie to you, this suture is tricky, but it's really satisfying when it works well. This suture is useful for straight wounds, is usually performed with an absorbable suture, and gives an 'invisible stitch' result.

We start at one edge of the wound. If you're right handed then start at the right, vice-versa for left handed. First, pass the needle deeply through one side of the wound, close to the corner. The needle starts off quite deep in the dermis and exits even deeper.

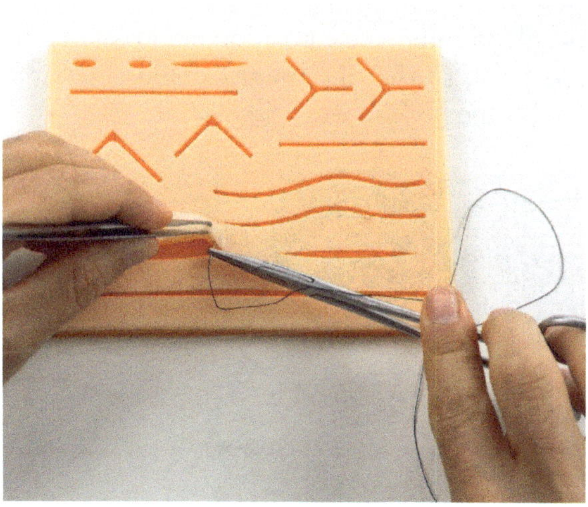

Tie a surgical knot and then cut the tail of the thread quite short (only leave around 2-3 mm).

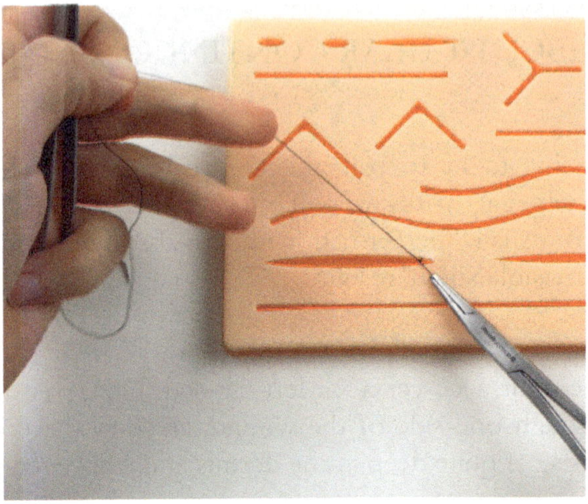

Place the needle in the reverse position, and pass the needle from deep to superficial, so that the point exits just below the surface and close to the apex of the wound.

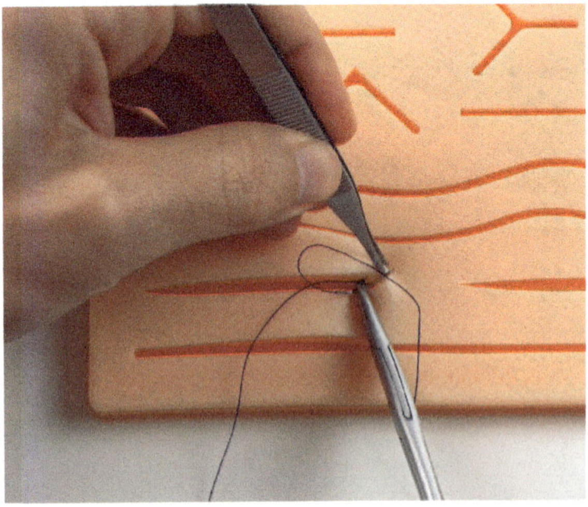

Now pass the needle through one side of the wound, travelling in a plane around 1-2 mm below the surface. Allow the needle to follow its curve.

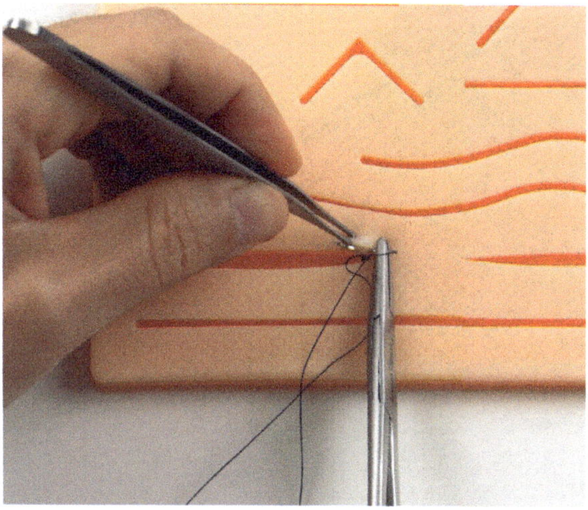

Reload the needle and repeat on the other side. Ensure your needle enters the skin directly opposite to where it has just exited.

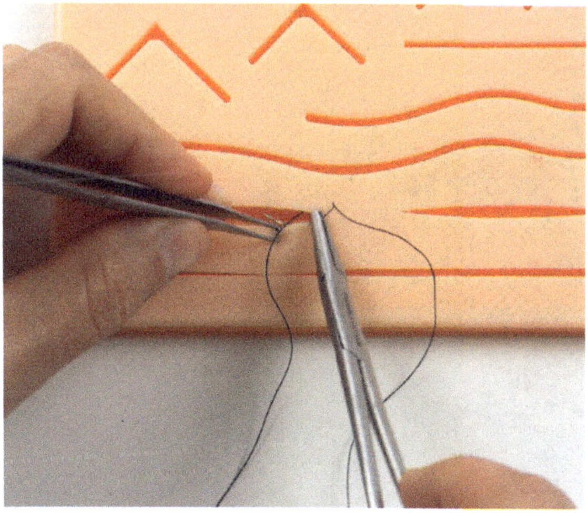

Keep repeating, gently pulling your thread tight as you go.

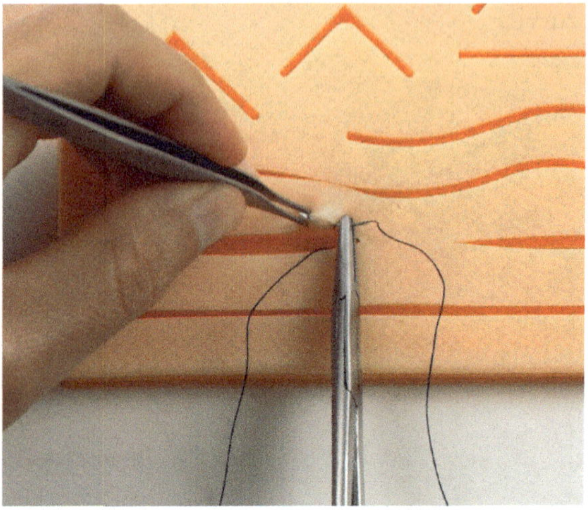

At the end of the wound, pass your needle from superficial to deep. Don’t pull the thread tight at this point, leave the loop of thread loose.

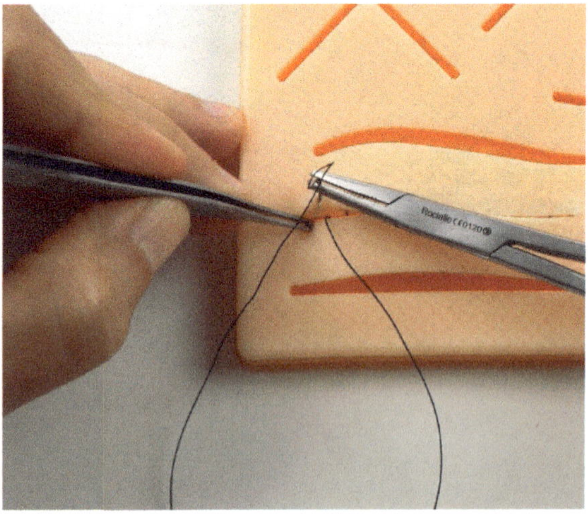

We can now tie off the suture, using an Aberdeen knot.
Keeping the thread under slight tension, place your other hand through the loop to grasp the thread.

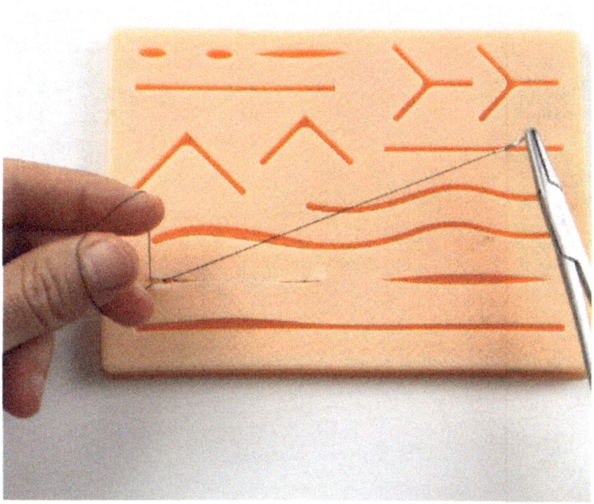

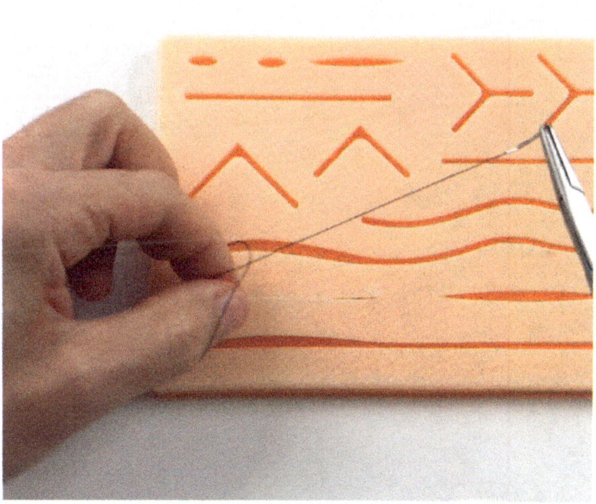

Pull this back through the loop, snugging the tie down.

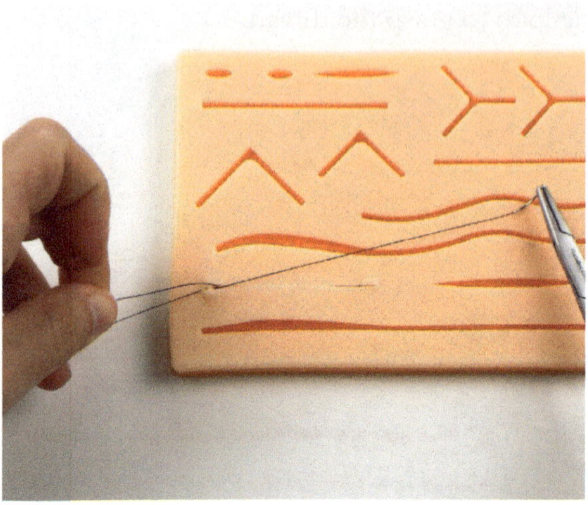

Repeat this step, pulling the thread back through the loop and again snugging the throw down.

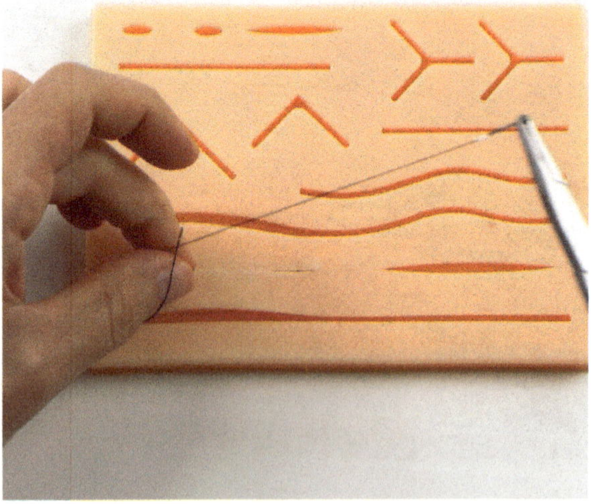

Then, pass the needle back through the loop and pull on the thread to lock the throw down and form a knot.

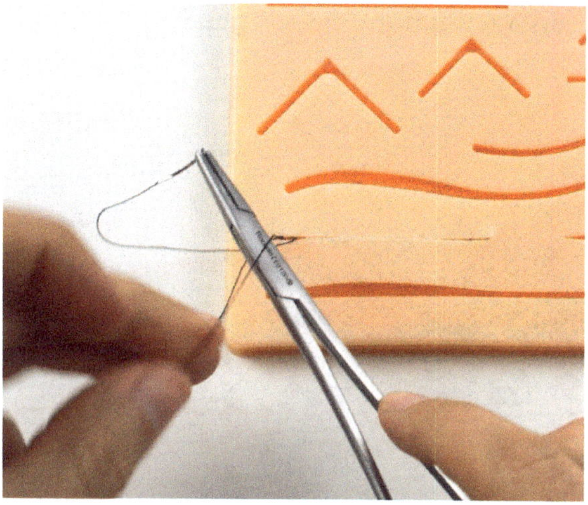

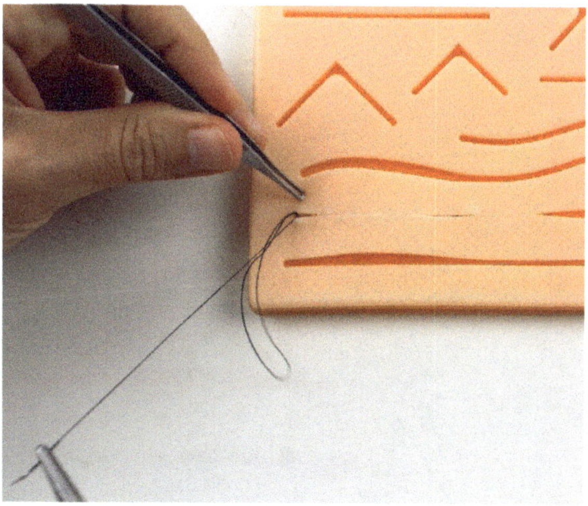

Finally, we are going to 'bury the knot' to reduce the chances of it spitting out. Pass your needle point just behind the knot and into the deep aspect of the wound. Feed your needle through so that the point exits a few mm from the wound.

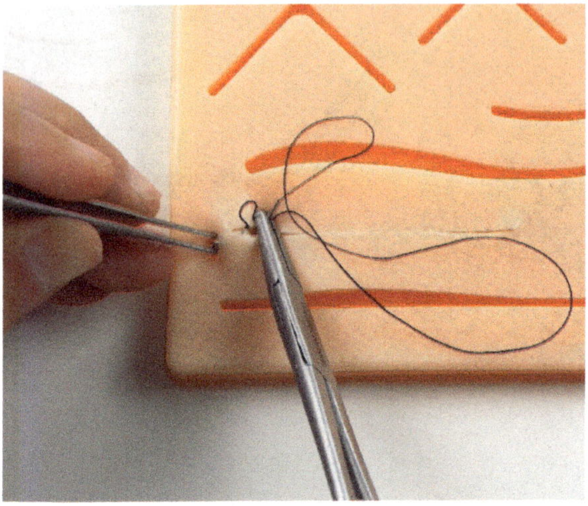

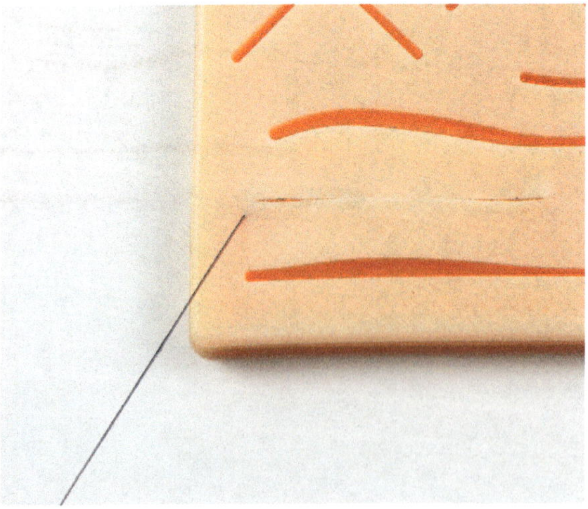

The thread can now be trimmed flush to the skin.

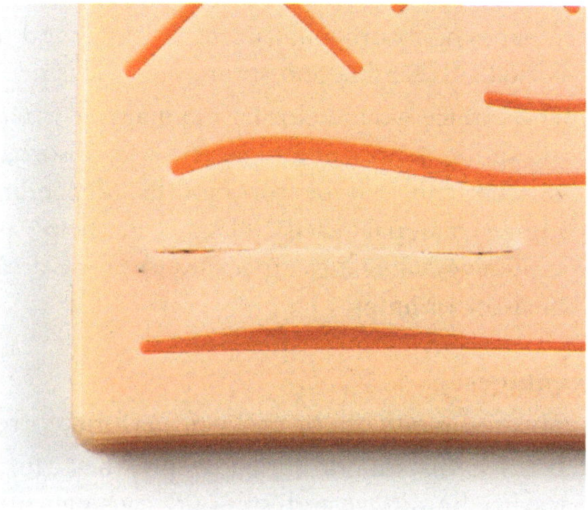

When you practice this suture, pull the wound edges apart to see the underlying pattern. Hopefully, you will see a 'train-track' appearance of the thread weaving in and out of the wound edges.

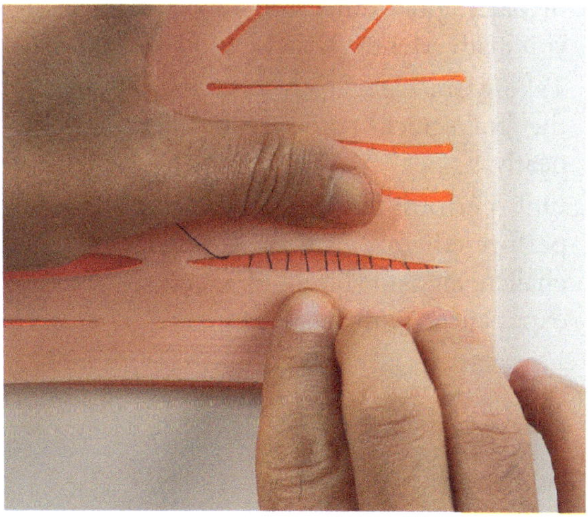

Advantages:

- As the suture runs in the dermis, there is no risk of poorer scarring due to 'suture marks'.
- When an absorbable suture is used and the knots buried as described, no suture removal is needed.
- The surface wound closure maintains its strength while the suture is present and intact; if an absorbable suture is used, this can be for months (depending on the suture material used). This can help avoid scar stretching/widening, especially in prone areas such as the back or limbs.

Disadvantages:

- This technique can be tricky to perform correctly.
- If the knots are not buried deeply, they can work their way to the surface and 'spit out', causing irritation.
- As this is a single thread, failure/breaking of any part can result in the entire wound dehiscing.

Top tips:

- Use a clear suture; as the thread travels in the more superficial parts of the dermis, a dyed suture (eg black or blue) could otherwise be visible through the skin if you inadvertently pass too close to the surface.
- Take extra care when passing your needle, to create the 'train-track' pattern, or the wound will not close neatly.
- Only perform this on a straight wound; whilst it can be performed on curved wounds, this is technically challenging and should be saved for when you are very experienced with this technique.

13 HALF-BURIED HORIZONTAL MATTRESS SUTURE

We've learnt the sutures most commonly used in skin surgery, so we can now turn to some neat suturing tricks that can really enhance your results. We've seen the horizontal mattress suture and the subcuticular suture – let's now combine the two.

First, we pass the needle as we would for a standard interrupted suture, but on one side only.

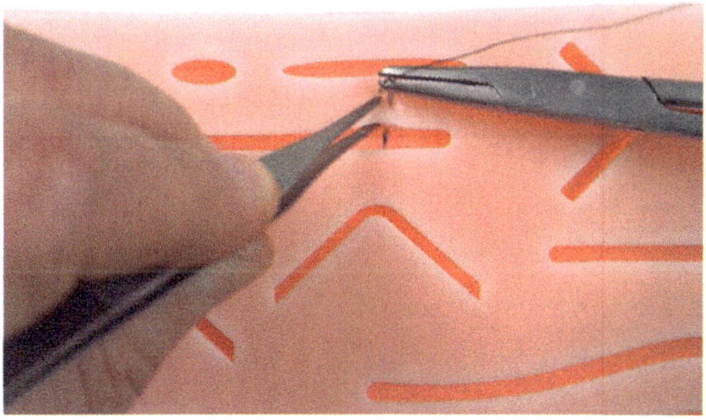

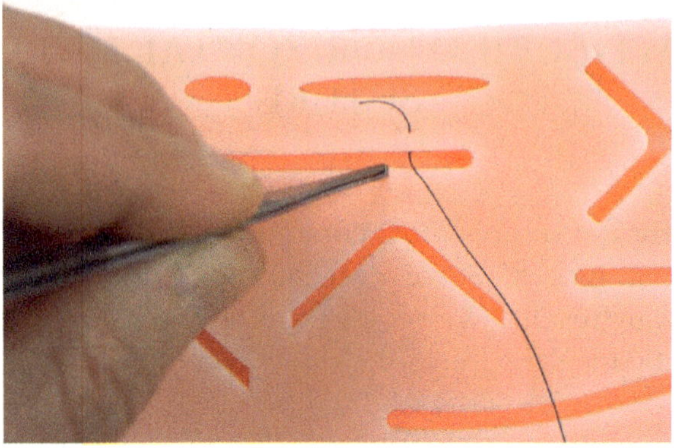

We now pass the needle through the dermis of the opposite wound edge. To do this, the needle enters the opposite dermis at the same depth that it exited from the first pass. Take a 'bite' of about 4-5mm of dermis, keeping at the same depth.

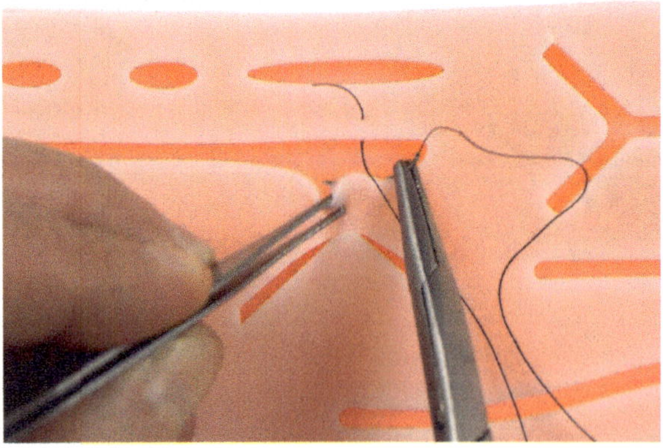

The needle is now passed back through the first edge, again at the same depth.

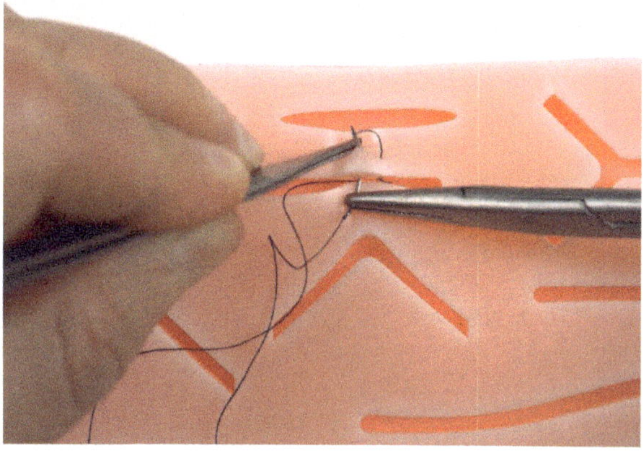

We can now tie the suture, using a standard instrument tie.

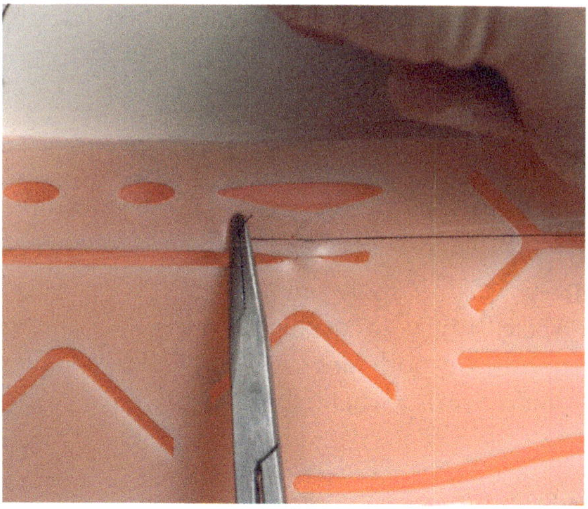

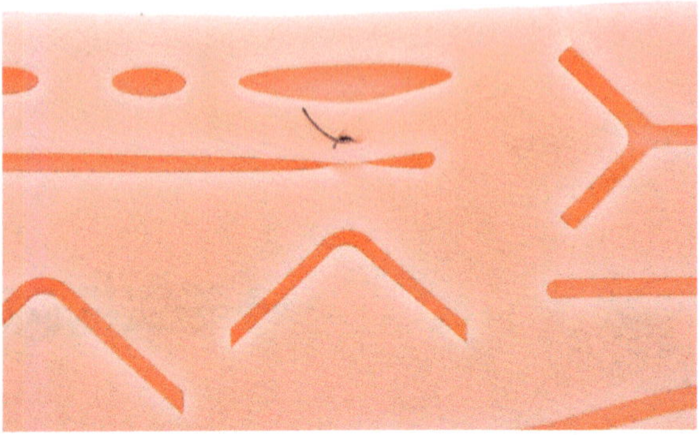

Advantages:

- The buried part runs in the dermis, so avoids the risk of 'stitch mark' scars.
- This is a useful technique when closing specific anatomical areas, such as the cleft where the cheek meets the base of the nose.

Disadvantages:

- This takes more time than a simple interrupted suture.

Top tips:

- Make sure your needle travels in the same depth of dermis on both sides of the wound, or the skin edges could overlap when closed.

14 THE CORNER SUTURE

As a Plastic surgeon, this suture is used fairly commonly when performing skin flaps. It is, though, also a really useful suture to know for when you have an irregular 'V' shaped wound or even a 'Y' shaped wound; these are commonly seen in the emergency room when faced with glass lacerations or other traumatic injuries.

When faced with a 'V' shaped wound, performing 3 or 4 standard sutures at, and around, the tip of the 'V' could potentially cause necrosis of the tip due to reduction in blood flow. We therefore want to try and avoid the strangulating effect of lots of sutures going into a small area, and this is where the corner suture can help.

We start by passing a suture through the skin opposite to the 'V', just lateral to the midline. The needle point exits at the depth of the dermis.

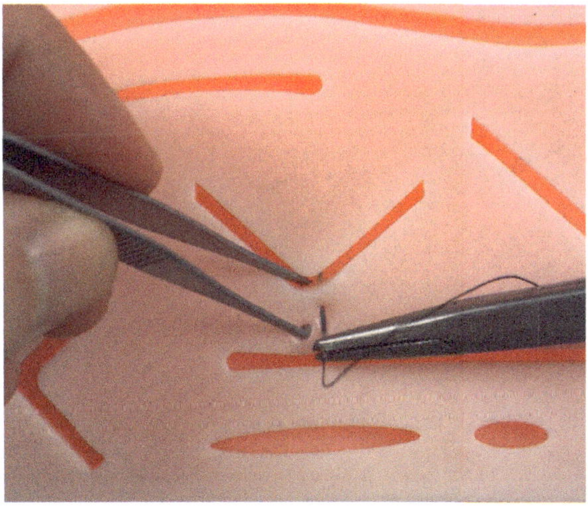

The needle is now passed through the tip of the 'V', passing at the same depth within the dermis.

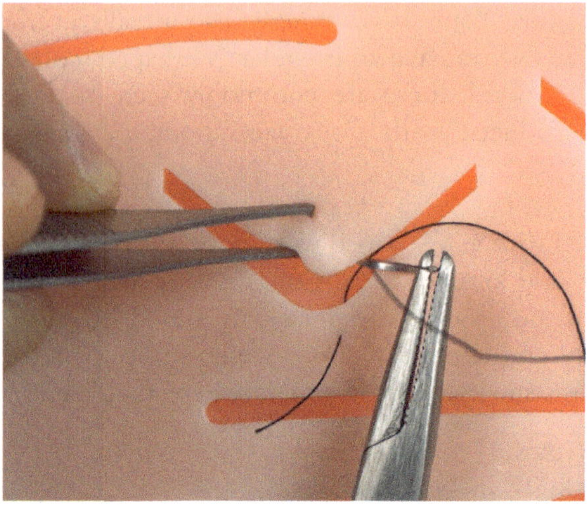

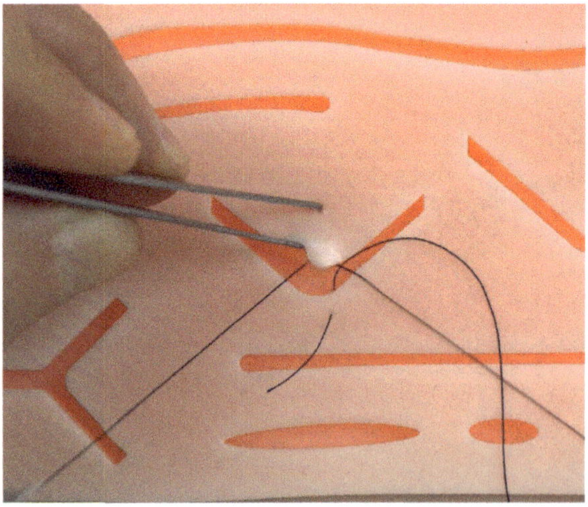

Then pass the needle back to the opposite skin edge, again entering the dermis at the same depth.

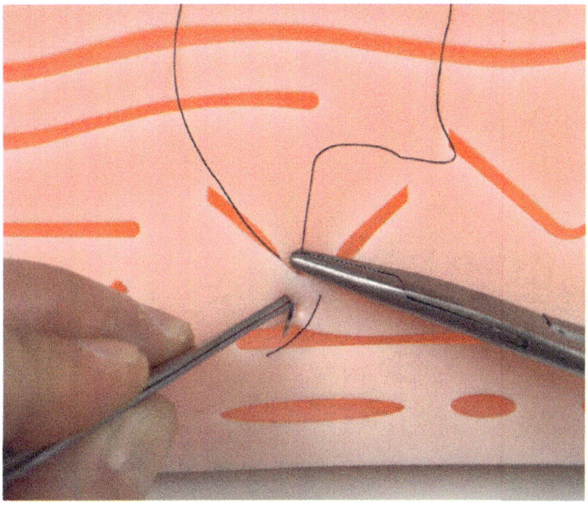

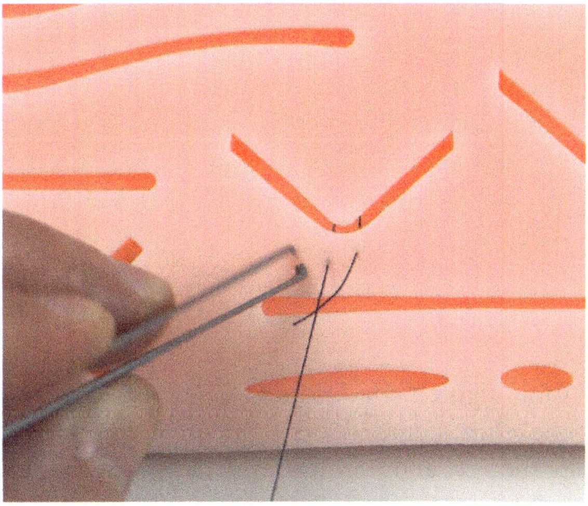

The suture can now be tied off, using our instrument tie.

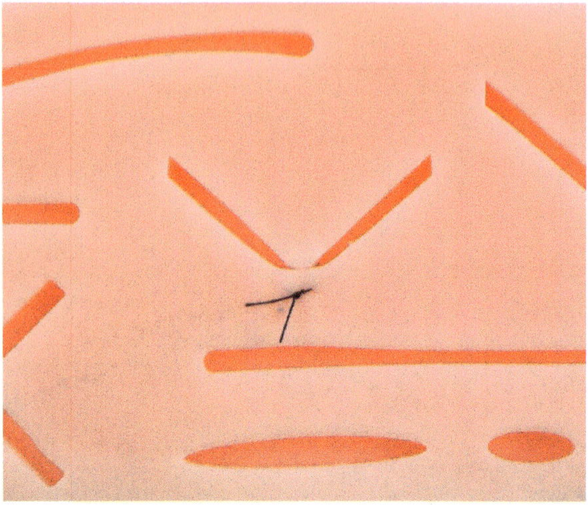

Advantages:

- This suture allows a 'V' shaped wound, such as seen in a flap or traumatic wound, to be closed with less suture material. This helps improve scarring.
- Having less sutures around the tip of the flap will reduce the chances of impaired blood flow and tissue necrosis.

Top tips:

- Only tighten the knots enough to gently approximate the skin edges; over-tightening can strangulate the tissue and lead to tissue necrosis.

15 CORNER SUTURE – ADVANCED TECHNIQUE

Having performed the corner suture for a 'V' shaped wound, what about a 'Y' shaped wound?

The principles are fairly similar, but with a slight difference – when we tie the suture, it is going to close part of the wound in the same way an interrupted suture would.

Pass the needle through one side of the wound, approximately 4-5 mm from the skin edge. The needle point exits at the depth of the dermis and should be heading towards one side of the 'V' apex.

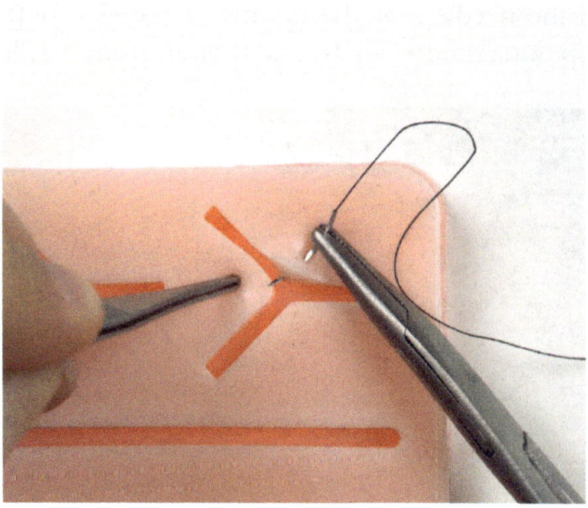

The needle now passes through the apex of the 'V' at the same dermal depth.

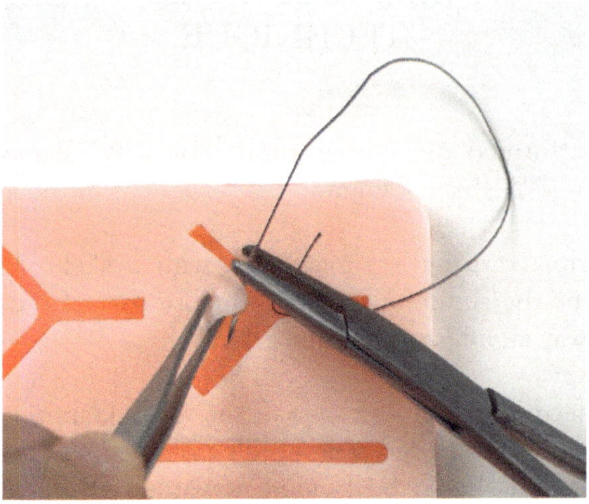

Now pass the needle into the dermis of the skin opposite your first entry point. Aim to exit around 4-5mm from the skin edge.

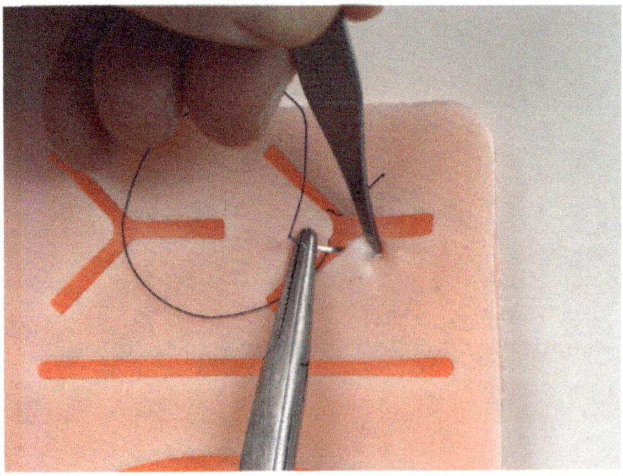

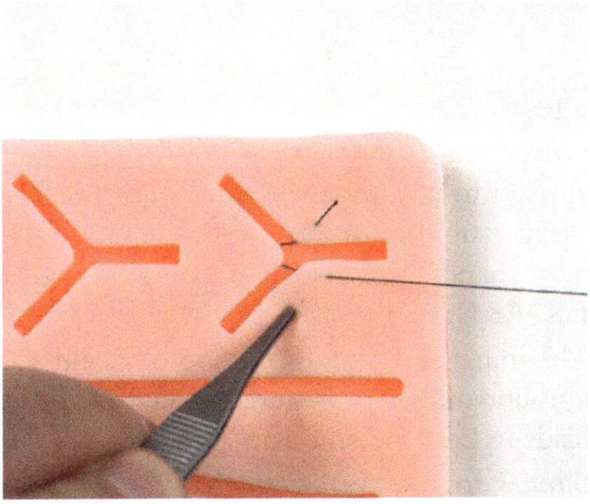

We're now ready to tie the suture. As you tighten your first throw, you will see the three points coming together; tighten enough to oppose the edges (bring them together), but as with all suturing, take care to not over-tighten. The rest of the wound can then be closed with interrupted sutures. You can see that a single suture has given the same result as 3 interrupted sutures, but with less trauma/suturing and risk of strangulation to the tip of the 'V'.

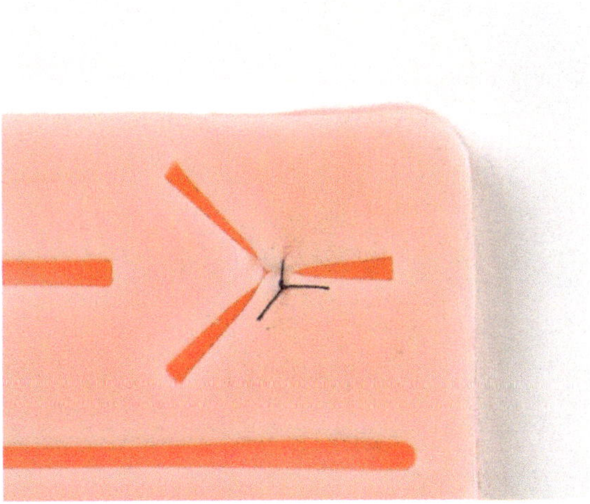

Advantages:

- Once you have mastered this technique it can be applied to a number of situations. Whilst it is used in Plastic surgery for closure of certain flaps, this is also very handy for closing complex wounds in the ER/A&E.
- The initial suture does the job of 3 and so reduces the amount of suture material placed in the wound. This leads to better cosmesis.
- Similar to the corner stitch, this technique gives the flap tip a greater chance of survival.

Disadvantages:

- It can be tricky to place the suture correctly, so does take some practice.

Top tips:

- Only tighten the knots enough to gently approximate the skin edges as over-tightening can increase the risk of flap tip necrosis.

16 - DEVELOPING YOUR SKILLS

As well as practicing on a suture pad, there are other ways to further develop your skills. Chicken breast can give a more realistic feel for suturing, whereas bananas are an economical way to practice. As a banana ripens, you will find that the skin becomes thinner and more friable, increasing the difficulty – grasp the edges too hard or pull the needle roughly and the skin will tear; this really helps to develop your tissue handling skills and needle technique.

Once you start to suture real skin, keep looking for any way to improve your technique. Is the result as neat as it could be? Are the knots nice and tight or looking too loose? What could you do next time to make it even better?
When you see your patient post-operatively, is the scar looking as good as it could? If not, why not?
By constantly questioning ourselves and striving for perfection, we can be sure we are giving the best care we can.

And of course, to see how the suturing is performed in practice, we have our courses. These are entirely online and pre-filmed, so can be taken at home, in your own time, and at your own pace.
At the end of the 'Suturing Skills' course you also get a certificate that is badged by both the Royal College of Surgeons of Edinburgh, and BAPRAS (British Association of Plastic, Reconstructive & Aesthetic Surgeons). Just go to **www.surgeryskills.com** to learn more.

OUR COURSES

If you are keen to improve your skills, stand out from the crowd, and get certificates to build your CV/portfolio, then head to Surgeryskills.com and look at our courses. Taught by Mr Tehrani, these courses give you the rare chance to be taught by a world-renowned Consultant Plastic surgeon in the comfort of your own home and at your own pace!

Introduction to Surgery

Aimed at medical students and first year qualified doctors and nurses, this course will help relieve some of the stress of going into theatre for the first time. You will learn how to perform a hand-tied reef knot, tying at depth, the instruments used, keeping instruments sterile and much more.
We at Surgeryskills.com are committed to sharing skills with as many people as possible, and so as a special offer with this book, **use code 'IntroFree' to get it completely free!**

Basic Suturing Skills virtual course

This course takes you step-by-step through numerous suture techniques including interrupted, mattress, continuous and subcuticular sutures. Taught by Mr Tehrani, this pre-filmed course can be taken whenever you want and at your own pace. Once completed you get a certificate that is badged by the Royal College of Surgeons of Edinburgh and the British Association of Plastic, Reconstructive & Aesthetic surgeons.
As a special offer with this book, **use code 'Suture20' to get 20% off.**

Minor Procedures course

Performing Minor procedure surgery is a common requirement, and not only for surgeons. Physicians/medics, family doctors and emergency care doctors and nurses are often faced with performing skin surgery and this course helps take the stress out of this. You will learn how to take biopsies, mark out excision margins, excise lesions, remove cysts, treat abscesses and more. This is again taught by our expert Plastic surgeon, Mr Tehrani, giving tips & tricks to get the best results and give the best care you can. It is also entirely online, so can be taken when you want and at your own leisure.

As a special offer with this book, **use code 'Procedure20' to get 20% off.**

(Unfortunately, we can only continue these offers while funding allows and so may end at any time)

We hope you've enjoyed reading this book and wish you the best of luck with your future career!

Surgery Skills

Learn Develop Excel

NOTES

Made in United States
North Haven, CT
10 November 2026

22088888R00055